Eula Biss is the auth ̃ ̃ ̃ ̃ ̃ ̃ ̃ ̃ ̃ ̃ ̃ ̃ ̃ ̃ ̃ of
the 10 Best Books of
From No Man's Land,
Critics Circle Awar<
Balloonists. Her work
York Times, The Belie٦
supported by an NE
Foundation Fellows١٦

'Imagine Eula Biss as herself a vaccine against vague and incoherent thinking, as a booster to the acuity of your thought, as a thermometer taking the temperature of our ideas about purity, contagion, individuality, and community. This book is a magnificent piece of research and of writing.'
— Rebecca Solnit, author of *Wanderlust*

'Like so many great nonfiction classics, *On Immunity* will teach, provoke, chafe, inspire, haunt, and likely change its many readers. Its central, difficult, and ecstatic premise – that 'we owe each other our bodies' – couldn't be more urgent, as the question of how we contend with this interdependence, this collectivity, is fundamental to our human present and future.'
— Maggie Nelson, author of *The Argonauts*

'Sontag said she wrote *Illness as Metaphor* to "calm the imagination, not to incite it," and *On Immunity* also seeks to cool and console. But where Sontag was imperious, Biss is stealthy. She advances from all sides, like a chess player, drawing on science, myth, literature to herd us to the only logical end, to vaccinate.'
— Parul Sehgal, *New York Times*

'*On Immunity* is brave because it will attract hostility from those she implies are selfish or misguided in refusing to vaccinate. Her arguments are profoundly compelling, and her narratives are braided together with beauty and elegance. The book is itself an inoculation – it grafts and unites different traditions of the essay, and in doing so creates something stronger and more resilient. And its urgent message is an inoculation against ignorance and fearmongering: may it spread out through the world, bringing substance and common sense to the vaccination debate.'
— Gavin Francis, *Guardian*

'*On Immunity* is as political as it is personal – Biss rails against a capitalism that has made unnatural individuals of us all – and as philosophical as it is political. ... What Biss does best, however, is doubt. She develops arguments and amasses detail but she also allows her writing to be shot through with uncertainty. Not often does a writer baldly admit that they don't know what something means (in this case, the ending of *Candide*). It is a very human non-fiction that emerges, comfortable with its questions.'
—— Sophie Elmhirst, *Financial Times*

'Eula Biss accomplishes two remarkable things in this book. She efficiently dismantles the wall between self-documentation and world-documentation. And she synthesizes a vast amount of information into the haunting and inescapable conclusion that "we are ... continuous with everything here on earth, including – and especially – each other."'
—— Sarah Manguso, author of *Ongoing*

'If you are yourself a nonfiction author, your initial response to this book might be to decide immediately on another line of work; Biss is that intimidatingly talented. This is cultural commentary at its highest level.'
—— *Washington Post*

'*On Immunity* casts a spell. ... There's a drama in watching this smart writer feel her way through this material. She's a poet, an essayist, and a class spy. She digs honestly into her own psyche and into those of "people like me", and she reveals herself as believer and apostate, moth and flame.'
——Dwight Garner, *New York Times*

Fitzcarraldo Editions
8-12 Creekside
London, SE8 3DX
United Kingdom

This first paperback edition published
by Fitzcarraldo Editions in 2020

ISBN 978-1-913097-40-0

Design by Ray O'Meara
Typeset in Fitzcarraldo
Printed and bound by CPI Group (UK) Ltd

fitzcarraldoeditions.com

On Immunity
An Inoculation

For other mothers, *with gratitude to mine*

¶ The first story I ever heard about immunity was told to me by my father, a doctor, when I was very young. It was the myth of Achilles, whose mother tried to make him immortal. She burned away his mortality with fire, in one telling of the story, and Achilles was left impervious to injury everywhere except his heel, where a poisoned arrow would eventually wound and kill him. In another telling, the infant Achilles was immersed in the River Styx, the river that divides the world from the underworld. His mother held her baby by his heel to dip him in the water, leaving, again, one fatal vulnerability.

When Rubens painted the life of Achilles, the River Styx is where he began. Bats fly across the sky of that painting and the dead ride a ferry in the distance. Achilles dangles from his mother's hand by one plump leg, with his head and shoulders entirely underwater. This is clearly no ordinary bath. The three-headed hound who guards the underworld lies curled at the base of the painting where the baby's body meets the river, as if the baby is being plunged into the beast. Conferring immunity, the painting suggests, is a perilous task.

To prepare her children for the hazards of life, my own mother read Grimms' fairy tales aloud to us every night before bed. I do not remember the brutality for which those tales are famous as vividly as I remember their magic—the golden pears growing in the castle garden, the boy no bigger than a thumb, the twelve brothers who became twelve swans. But it did not escape my notice, as a child, that the parents in those tales have a maddening habit of getting tricked into making bad gambles with their children's lives.

In one story, a man agrees to trade with the devil whatever is standing beyond his mill. He thinks he is giving away his apple tree, but to his dismay he finds his daughter standing beyond the mill. In another story, a woman who has been longing for a child becomes pregnant and craves a plant called Rapunzel that grows in the garden of a wicked enchantress. The woman sends her husband to steal the plant and when he is caught, he promises their future child to the enchantress, who locks the girl away in a tall tower with no door. But maidens locked in towers will let down their hair.

And so it was in the Greek myths my mother read to me later. A king who had heard an ominous prophecy could not keep his daughter childless by locking her in a tower. Zeus visited her in the form of a shower of gold that left her pregnant with a child who later killed the king. When the infant Oedipus, left on a mountainside to die, was saved by a shepherd, he was not saved from the prophecy that foretold he would kill his father and marry his mother. And Thetis, Achilles's mother, could neither burn nor drown his mortality.

A child cannot be kept from his fate, though this does not stop the gods themselves from trying. Achilles's mother, a goddess who married a mortal, heard a prophecy that her son would die young. She made every effort to defy this prophecy, including dressing Achilles as a girl during the Trojan War. After he took up a sword and was discovered to be a boy, his mother asked the god of fire to make a shield for him. This shield was emblazoned with the sun and moon, the earth and ocean, cities at war and peace, fields plowed and reaped—the universe, with all its dualities, was Achilles's shield.

The story my father told me when I was young was not the myth of Achilles, he reminds me now, but another ancient story. As my father relates the plot, I understand why I confused the two. The hero of this story is made immune to injury by bathing in the blood of a dragon. But a leaf clings to his body while he bathes, leaving a small spot on his back where he is unprotected. After having been victorious in many battles, he is killed by one blow to that spot.

Immunity is a myth, these stories suggest, and no mortal can ever be made invulnerable. The truth of this was much easier for me to grasp before I became a mother. My son's birth brought with it an exaggerated sense of both my own power and my own powerlessness. I found myself bargaining with fate so frequently that my husband and I made a game of it, asking each other what disease we would give our child for prevention against another—a parody of the impossible decisions of parenthood.

When my son was an infant, I would hear many variations of "All that matters is that he is safe." I would wonder whether that was, indeed, all that mattered nearly as often as I would wonder if I could keep him safe. I was certain that I did not have the power to protect him from his fate, whatever it might be. But I was determined nonetheless to avoid the bad gambles of the Grimms' tales. I would not let my child be cursed by my own carelessness or cupidity. I would not accidentally say to the devil, *You may have what is beyond the mill*, only to discover that what is standing beyond the mill is my child.

¶ The day before my son was born was the first warm day of spring. In labor, I walked out to the end of the pier, where the morning sun was breaking up the ice floes on Lake Michigan. My husband held up a video camera and asked me to speak to the future, but the sound did not record, so whatever I said has been lost to the past. What remains evident on my face is that I was not afraid. During the long labor that followed that sunlit moment I imagined myself swimming in the lake, which became, against my will, a lake of darkness and then a lake of fire and then a lake without a horizon. By the time my son was born late the next day a cold rain was falling and I had crossed over into a new realm in which I was no longer fearless.

That spring, a novel strain of influenza would begin spreading from Mexico to the United States to the rest of the world. I did not register those early reports, as I was too busy listening to my son breathe at night. During the day, I was entirely preoccupied by how much he did or did not nurse, and how much he did or did not sleep. I cannot now decipher the entries I made in a notebook then—long lists of times, some of them only minutes apart. Obscure notations next to the times indicate, I think, waking, sleeping, nursing, and crying. I was searching for a pattern, trying to determine what made my baby cry inconsolably. What made him cry, I would learn much later, was an intolerance to cow's milk. Offending proteins from the milk I drank passed through my milk to him—a possibility that had not occurred to me.

By the end of the summer, the evening news was running footage of people wearing white surgical masks in airports. The novel influenza virus was officially pandemic at that point. Churches were serving holy wafers on toothpicks, and airlines were removing pillows and blankets from their flights. What surprises me now is how unremarkable this seemed to me at the time. It all became part of the landscape of new motherhood, where ordinary objects like pillows and blankets have the power to kill a newborn. Colleges were daily sterilizing every "high-touch" surface, while I was nightly boiling every object my child put in his mouth. It was as if the nation had joined me in the paranoia of infant care. Like many other mothers, I had been informed of a syndrome affecting infants that had no warning signs and no symptoms other than sudden death. Perhaps this is why, despite everything, I do not remember feeling particularly scared of the flu—it was just one concern of many. There was lead paint, I knew, on my walls and hexavalent chromium in my water, and the books I was reading were telling me to run a fan while my baby slept because even stagnant air could suffocate him.

When I search now for a synonym for *protect*, my thesaurus suggests, after *shield* and *shelter* and *secure*, one final option: *inoculate*. This was the question, when my son was born—would I inoculate him? As I understood it then, this was not a question of whether I would protect him so much as it was a question of whether inoculation was a risk worth taking. Would I enter into a gamble, like Thetis dipping the infant Achilles into the River Styx?

The mothers I knew began debating whether or not to vaccinate our children against the novel influenza virus long before any vaccine became available to us. We were hearing that what made this particular strain of flu dangerous was that it was new to humans, like the virus that caused the Spanish flu epidemic of 1918 in which more than 50 million people died. But then we were also hearing that the vaccine had been produced hurriedly and that it might not have been fully tested.

One mother told us that she had miscarried while she was sick with the seasonal flu and, being wary of any flu now, she planned to vaccinate. Another mother said that her child had screamed frighteningly all night following her first vaccination and she would not risk another vaccination of any kind. Every exchange about the new flu vaccine was an extension of the already existing discussion about immunization, in which all that is known of disease is weighed against all that is unknown about vaccines.

As the virus spread, a mother I knew in Florida reported that her entire family had just had the H1N1 flu and it was not any worse than a bad cold. Another mother in Chicago told me that her friend's healthy nineteen-year-old son had suffered a stroke after being hospitalized with the flu. I believed both of these stories, but they told me nothing more than what the Centers for Disease Control and Prevention already seemed to be trying to tell me—the flu could be harmless in some cases and serious in others. Under the circumstances, vaccination began to seem prudent. My baby was just over six months old and I had just returned to work at a large university where the majority of my students would be coughing by the last week of classes.

That fall, the *New Yorker* ran an article in which Michael Specter noted that influenza is regularly among the top ten causes of death in the United States and that even relatively mild pandemics of influenza have killed in the millions. "And, though this H1N1 virus is novel," he wrote, "the vaccine is not. It was made and tested in exactly the same way that flu vaccines are always made and tested." Some of the mothers I knew did not like the tone of this article. They found it insulting for the same reason I found it reassuring—it did not acknowledge any good reason for doubt.

The fact that the press is an unreliable source of information was one of the refrains of my conversations with other mothers, along with the fact that the government is inept, and that big pharmaceutical companies are corrupting medicine. I agreed with all these concerns, but I was disturbed by the worldview they suggested: nobody can be trusted.

It was not a good season for trust. The United States was engaged in two ongoing wars that seemed to be benefiting no one other than military contractors. People were losing their houses and their jobs while the government was bailing out the financial institutions it deemed too big to fail and using taxpayer money to shore up the banks. It did not seem unlikely that our government favored the interests of corporations over the well-being of its citizens.

During the initial aftershocks of the economic crash there was talk of "restoring the public's trust," though even then the emphasis fell more often than not on consumer confidence. I disliked the term *consumer confidence*, and I bristled every time I was encouraged to trust myself as a mother. I had little confidence, consumer or otherwise, but I tended to believe that confidence was less important than the kind of trust that transcends the self. Even now, years after my son's birth, I remain interested in the precise meaning of *trust*, particularly in legal and financial terms. A trust—in the sense of a valuable asset placed in the care of someone to whom it does not ultimately belong—captures, more or less, my understanding of what it is to have a child.

By late October, the mothers who were still talking about the flu vaccine were mainly talking about how hard it was to get a child vaccinated. My son had been on a waiting list at his pediatrician's office for over a month. Other mothers were waiting in long lines outside community colleges and public high schools. While we waited, a mother who did not vaccinate her children mentioned that she had heard there was an additive called squalene in the H1N1 vaccine. No, another mother countered, squalene was used in flu vaccines in Europe, but it was not used here. The mother who had originally mentioned squalene was not so sure—the fact that US vaccines did not contain squalene, she said, had been disputed elsewhere. "Where exactly is elsewhere?" one of my friends wondered. *What*, I wondered, *is squalene?*

The women with whom I debated the merits of the flu vaccine possessed a technical vocabulary that was entirely unfamiliar to me at the time. They used words like *adjuvant* and *conjugate*, and they knew which vaccines were live virus vaccines and which were acellular. They were familiar with the intricacies of the vaccine schedules of other countries, and literate in an array of vaccine additives. Many of them were, like me, writers. And so it is not surprising that I began to hear metaphors behind the technical language and information we traded.

Squalene is found in a great many living things including the human body, where it is manufactured in the liver. It circulates in our blood and is left behind in our fingerprints. Some European flu vaccines do indeed contain squalene from shark liver oil, but squalene has never been added to US-licensed vaccines. Squalene's presence in absence is something like the curious properties of thimerosal, the mercury-based preservative that was removed from every childhood vaccine except multi-dose flu vaccines by 2002. Well over a decade later, fear of mercury in vaccines persists.

My son finally got his flu vaccination in late November. We didn't know it yet, but the worst of the pandemic was already over—cases of H1N1 influenza had peaked in October. I remember asking the nurse if the vaccine my son was receiving contained thimerosal, but I was asking more out of due diligence than true concern. I already suspected that if there was a problem with vaccines it was not thimerosal, and it was not squalene.

¶ "What's that?" was my son's first phrase, and for a long time it was all he could say. As he learned to talk, I learned, in naming the parts of things for him, how often our language reflects our bodies. "We give a chair arms, legs, a seat and a back," writes the poet Marvin Bell, "a cup has its lip / and a bottle its neck." The ability to make and understand basic metaphors of this kind arrives with language, which is itself made of metaphor. Plumbing almost any word will reveal what Emerson called "fossil poetry," metaphors submerged below the surface of our current usage. *Fathom*, a means of measuring the depth of the ocean, now means *understand* because its literal origin, using outstretched arms to measure cloth from fingertip to fingertip, was once used as a metaphor for grasping an idea.

"Our bodies prime our metaphors," writes James Geary in *I Is an Other*, his treatise on metaphor, "and our metaphors prime how we think and act." If we source our understanding of the world from our own bodies, it seems inevitable that vaccination would become emblematic: a needle breaks the skin, a sight so profound that it causes some people to faint, and a foreign substance is injected directly into the flesh. The metaphors we find in this gesture are overwhelmingly fearful, and almost always suggest violation, corruption, and pollution.

The British call it a "jab," and Americans, favoring guns, call it a "shot." Either way, vaccination is a violence. And when vaccination is intended to prevent a sexually transmitted disease, it seems to become a sexual violence. In 2011, Republican presidential candidate Michele Bachmann warned of the "ravages" of the vaccine against human papillomavirus and argued that is was wrong "to have innocent little twelve-year-old girls be forced to have a government injection." Her opponent Rick Santorum agreed, adding that no purpose was served by "having little girls innoculated at the force and compulsion of the government." The vaccine, some parents had already complained, was "inappropriate for girls of such a young age," and other parents feared it would encourage promiscuity.

Throughout the nineteenth century, vaccination left a wound that would scar. "The mark of the beast," some feared. In an Anglican archbishop's 1882 sermon, vaccination was akin to an injection of sin, an "abominable mixture of corruption, the lees of human vice, and dregs of venial appetites, that in after life may foam upon the spirit, and develop hell within, and overwhelm the soul."

While vaccination no longer leaves a mark in most cases, our fears that we will be permanently marked have remained. We fear that vaccination will invite autism or any one of the diseases of immune dysfunction that now plague industrialized countries—diabetes, asthma, and allergies. We fear that the hepatitis B vaccine will cause multiple sclerosis, or that the diphtheria-tetanus-pertussis vaccine will cause sudden infant death. We fear that the combination of several vaccines at once will tax the immune system, and that the total number of vaccines will overwhelm it. We fear that the formaldehyde in some vaccines will cause cancer, or that the aluminum in others will poison our brains.

It was "the poison of adders, the blood, entrails and excretions of rats, bats, toads and sucking whelps" that was imagined into vaccines of the nineteenth century. This was the kind of organic matter, the filth, believed responsible for most disease at that time. It was also a plausible recipe for a witches' brew. Vaccination was fairly dangerous then. Not because it would cause a child to grow the horns of a cow, as some people feared, but because arm-to-arm vaccination could communicate diseases like syphilis, as some people suspected. In arm-to-arm vaccination, the pus from the blister that developed on a recently vaccinated person's arm was used to vaccinate another person. Even after vaccination no longer involved an exchange of bodily fluids, bacterial contamination remained a problem. In 1901, a vaccine contaminated with tetanus bacteria killed nine children in Camden, New Jersey.

Now our vaccines are, if all is well, sterile. Some contain preservatives to prevent the growth of bacteria. So now it is, in the activist Jenny McCarthy's words, "the frickin' mercury, the ether, the aluminum, the antifreeze" that we fear in our vaccines. Our witches' brew is chemical. There is not actually any ether or antifreeze in vaccines, but these substances speak to anxieties about our industrial world. They evoke the chemicals on which we now blame our bad health, and the pollutants that now threaten our environment.

An 1881 handbill titled *The Vaccination Vampire* warns of the "universal pollution" delivered by the vaccinator to the "pure babe." Known to feed on the blood of babies, the vampires of that time became a ready metaphor for the vaccinators who inflicted wounds on infants. Blood-sucking monsters of ancient folklore were hideous, but Victorian vampires could be seductive. The macabre sexuality of the vampire dramatized the fear that there was something sexual in the act of vaccination, an anxiety that was only reinforced when sexually transmitted diseases were spread through arm-to-arm vaccination. Victorian vampires, like Victorian doctors, were associated not just with corruption of the blood, but also with economic corruption. Having virtually invented a paid profession and being almost exclusively available to the rich, doctors were suspect to the working class.

Bram Stoker's Count Dracula is of the bloodthirsty bourgeois—he keeps dusty piles of gold coins in his castle, and gold coins pour from his cloak when he is stabbed. But it is difficult to read him as a vaccinator. Of all the metaphors suggested within the plentiful pages of *Dracula*, disease is one of the most obvious. Dracula arrives in England just as a new disease might arrive, on a boat. He summons hoards of rats, and his infective evil spreads from the first woman he bites to the children she feeds on, unwittingly, at night. What makes Dracula particularly terrifying, and what takes the plot of the story so long to resolve, is that he is a monster whose monstrosity is contagious.

Germ theory was widely accepted by 1897, the year *Dracula* was published, but only after having been ridiculed earlier in the century. The suspicion that microorganisms of some sort caused disease had been around for so long that the theory was already considered outdated by the time Louis Pasteur demonstrated the presence of germs in the air with his corked and uncorked flasks of sterile broth. Among the vampire hunters who pursue Dracula, "sterilizing" his coffins so that he cannot take refuge in them, are two doctors, who initially disagree on their diagnosis. The younger doctor cannot bring himself to believe in vampires, despite the evidence, so the older doctor delivers an impassioned speech on the intersection of science and faith.

"Let me tell you, my friend," he says, "that there are things done today in electrical science which would have been deemed unholy by the very men who discovered electricity—who would themselves not so long before have been burned as wizards." He then goes on to evoke Mark Twain: "I heard once of an American who so defined faith: 'that which enables us to believe things which we know to be untrue,'" saying, "He meant that we shall have an open mind, and not let a little bit of truth check the rush of a big truth, like a small rock does a railway truck."

Dracula is as much about this problem, the problem of evidence and truth, as it is about vampires. In proposing that one truth may derail another, it invites an enduring question—do we believe vaccination to be more monstrous than disease?

¶ "Deep within every man there lies the dread of being alone in the world, forgotten by God, overlooked among the tremendous household of millions upon millions," Søren Kierkegaard wrote in his journal in 1847. That was the year he finished *Works of Love*, in which he insists that love is known not through words, but only "by its fruits."

I read the first fifty pages of *Works of Love* in college before giving it up out of exhaustion. In those pages Kierkegaard unfolds the commandment "You shall love your neighbor as yourself," parsing it almost word by word, so that after exploring the nature of love he asks what is meant by "as yourself," and then what is meant by "your neighbor," and then what is meant by "you shall." Overwhelmed, I stopped reading shortly after Kierkegaard asked, *"Who, then, is one's neighbor?,"* which he answered, in part, with, *"Neighbor* is what philosophers would call the *other,* that by which the selfishness in self-love is to be tested." I had read enough at that point to be troubled by the idea that one must enact one's beliefs, and perhaps even embody them.

From somewhere deep in my childhood I can remember my father explaining with enthusiasm the principle behind the Doppler effect as an ambulance sped past our car. When we watched the sun set over the river where we lived he described Rayleigh scattering, the removal of the shorter wavelengths of light by the atmosphere that results in reddish clouds and grass that looks more intensely green at dusk. In the woods he dissected an owl pellet for me, and reassembled from it the tiny skeleton of a mouse. My father marveled at the natural world far more often than he talked about the human body, but blood types were a subject on which he spoke with some passion.

People with the blood type O negative, he explained, can only receive in transfusion blood that is O negative, but people with O-negative blood can give blood to people of any other type. That's why a person with Type O negative is known as a "universal donor." My father would then reveal that his blood type was O negative, that he himself was a universal donor. He gave blood, my father explained, as often as he was allowed because blood of his type was always in demand for emergency transfusions. I suspect my father may have already known then what I would only discover later—that my blood, too, is Type O negative.

I understood the universal donor more as an ethic than as a medical concept long before I knew my own blood type. But I did not yet think of that ethic as an ingenious filtering of my father's Catholicism through his medical training. I was not raised in the Church and I never took communion, so I was not reminded of Jesus offering his blood that we all might live when my father spoke of the universal donor. But I believed, even then, that we owe each other our bodies.

Every time my father went out in a boat, for my entire childhood, he took a life preserver with his name and "Organ Donor" printed hugely on it in permanent ink. It was a joke in which he believed quite sincerely. When he taught me to drive, he gave me this advice from his own father: you are responsible not just for the car you are driving, but also for the car ahead of you and the car behind you. Learning to drive all three cars was daunting, and inspired an occasional paralysis that plagues driving to this day, but when I earned my license I signed my name under Organ Donor.

The very first decision I made for my son, a decision enacted within moments of his body coming free of mine, was the donation of his umbilical cord blood to a public bank. At thirty, I had only donated blood once, back in college when I was reading Kierkegaard. I wanted my son to start his life with a credit to the bank, not the debt I already felt. And this was before I, a universal donor, would become the sole recipient of two units of blood in transfusion after my son's birth—blood of the most precious type, drawn from a public bank.

If we imagine the action of a vaccine not just in terms of how it affects a single body, but also in terms of how it affects the collective body of a community, it is fair to think of vaccination as a kind of banking of immunity. Contributions to this bank are donations to those who cannot or will not be protected by their own immunity. This is the principle of *herd immunity*, and it is through herd immunity that mass vaccination becomes far more effective than individual vaccination.

Any given vaccine can fail to produce immunity in an individual, and some vaccines, like the influenza vaccine, are less effective than others. But when enough people are vaccinated with even a relatively ineffective vaccine, viruses have trouble moving from host to host and cease to spread, sparing both the unvaccinated and those in whom vaccination has not produced immunity. This is why the chances of contracting measles can be higher for a vaccinated person living in a largely unvaccinated community than they are for an unvaccinated person living in a largely vaccinated community.

The unvaccinated person is protected by the bodies around her, bodies through which disease is not circulating. But a vaccinated person surrounded by bodies that host disease is left vulnerable to vaccine failure or fading immunity. We are protected not so much by our own skin, but by what is beyond it. The boundaries between our bodies begin to dissolve here. Donations of blood and organs move between us, exiting one body and entering another, and so too with immunity, which is a common trust as much as it is a private account. Those of us who draw on collective immunity owe our health to our neighbors.

When my son was six months old, at the peak of the H1N1 flu pandemic, another mother told me that she did not believe in herd immunity. It was only a theory, she said, and one that applied mainly to cows. That herd immunity was subject to belief had not yet occurred to me, though there is clearly something of the occult in the idea of an invisible cloak of protection cast over the entire population.

Aware that I did not fully understand the mechanism behind this magic, I searched the university library for articles about herd immunity. As early as 1840, I learned, a doctor observed that vaccinating only part of a population against smallpox could arrest an epidemic in full. This indirect protection from disease could also be observed, temporarily, after large numbers of people acquired natural immunity from infection during an epidemic. In the era before vaccination against childhood diseases like measles, epidemics tended to come in waves followed by lulls during which the number of new children who had not been made immune by infection crept toward some crucial, but unknown, proportion of the population. Herd immunity, an observable phenomenon, now seems implausible only if we think of our bodies as inherently disconnected from other bodies. Which, of course, we do.

The very expression herd immunity suggests that we are cattle, waiting, perhaps, to be sent to slaughter.

And it invites an unfortunate association with the term *herd mentality*, a stampede toward stupidity. The herd, we assume, is foolish. Those of us who eschew the herd mentality tend to prefer a frontier mentality in which we imagine our bodies as isolated homesteads that we tend either well or badly. The health of the homestead next to ours does not affect us, this thinking suggests, so long as ours is well tended.

If we were to exchange the metaphor of the herd for a hive, perhaps the concept of shared immunity might be more appealing. Honeybees are matriarchal, environmental do-gooders who also happen to be entirely interdependent. The health of any individual bee, as we know from the recent epidemic of colony collapse, depends on the health of the hive. In *The Wisdom of Crowds*, journalist James Surowiecki details the sophisticated scouting and reporting methods honeybees use to gather nectar. The cooperative work of bees, Surowiecki suggests, is an example of the kind of collective problem solving our own society depends on.

While there are many well-documented instances of crowds making bad decisions—lynching comes to mind—Surowiecki observes that large groups routinely solve complex problems that evade individuals. Groups of people, if they are sufficiently diverse and free to disagree, can provide us with thinking superior to any one expert's. Groups can locate lost submarines, predict the stock market, and reveal the cause of a new disease. In March 2003, after a mysterious respiratory disease killed five people in China, the World Health Organization arranged a collaboration between research laboratories in ten different countries to identify the cause of what would come to be known as SARS. The labs, themselves made up of teams, worked together, sharing information and debating their results in daily conferences. By April, they had isolated the novel virus responsible for the disease. No one person had been in charge of the process, and no one person could claim credit for the discovery. Science, Surowiecki reminds us, is "a profoundly collective enterprise." It is a product of the herd.

¶ My son is fully vaccinated, but there is one immunization on the standard schedule that he did not receive on time. This was meant to be his very first shot, the hep B administered to most babies immediately after birth. In the months before my son was born, while I was teaching at the university and hauling a used crib through the snow and moving bookshelves to make room for the crib, I began spending my evenings reading articles about immunization. I was already aware, before I became pregnant, of some fears around vaccination. But I was not prepared for the labyrinthine network of interlocking anxieties I would discover during my pregnancy, the proliferation of hypotheses, the minutiae of additives, the diversity of ideologies.

Finding that the reach of my subject had far exceeded the limits of my late-night research by the time my baby was due, I visited the pediatrician I had chosen to be my son's doctor. A number of friends had offered his name when I asked for a recommendation, and so had my midwife, who referred to him as "left of center." When I asked the pediatrician what the purpose of the hep B vaccine was, he answered, "That's a very good question," in a tone that I understood to mean this was a question he relished answering. Hep B was a vaccine for the *inner city*, he told me, designed to protect the babies of drug addicts and prostitutes. It was not something, he assured me, that people like me needed to worry about.

All that this doctor knew of me then was what he could see. He assumed, correctly, that I did not live in the inner city. It did not occur to me to clarify for the doctor that although I live in the outer city of Chicago, my neighborhood is very much like what some people mean when they use the term *inner city*. In retrospect, I am ashamed by how little of his racial code I registered.

Relieved to be told that this vaccine was not for people like me, I failed to consider what exactly that meant.

The belief that public health measures are not intended for people like us is widely held by many people like me. Public health, we assume, is for people with less— less education, less-healthy habits, less access to quality health care, less time and money. I have heard mothers of my class suggest, for instance, that the standard childhood immunization schedule groups together multiple shots because poor mothers will not visit the doctor frequently enough to get the twenty-six recommended shots separately. No matter that any mother, myself included, might find so many visits daunting. *That*, we seem to be saying of the standard schedule, *is for people like them*.

In an article for *Mothering* magazine, the journalist Jennifer Margulis expresses outrage that newborn infants are routinely vaccinated against hep B and wonders why she was encouraged to vaccinate her daughter "against a sexually transmitted disease she had no chance of catching." Hep B is transmitted not only by sex, but through bodily fluids, so the most common way that infants contract hep B is from their mothers. Babies born to women who are infected with hep B—and mothers can carry the virus without their knowledge—will almost certainly be infected if they are not vaccinated within twelve hours of birth. The virus can also be passed through close contact between children, and people of any age can carry it without symptoms. Like human papillomavirus and a number of other viruses, hep B is a carcinogen, and it is most likely to cause cancer in people who contract it when they are young.

One of the mysteries of hep B immunization is that

vaccinating only "high risk" groups, which was the original public health strategy, did not bring down rates of infection. When the vaccine was introduced in 1981, it was recommended for prisoners, health care workers, gay men, and IV drug users. But rates of hep B infection remained unchanged until the vaccine was recommended for all newborns a decade later. Only mass vaccination brought down the rates of infection, and it has now virtually eliminated the disease in children.

The concept of a "risk group," Susan Sontag writes, "revives the archaic idea of a tainted community that illness has judged." Risk, in the case of hep B, turns out to be a rather complicated assessment. There is risk in having sex with just one partner, or traveling through the birth canal. In many cases, the source of infection is never known. I decided, before I knew how much blood I would lose in childbirth, that I did not want my son to be vaccinated against hep B. I did not belong to a risk group at the moment he was born, but by the time I put him to my breast I had received a blood transfusion and my status had changed.

When the last nationwide smallpox epidemic began in 1898, some people believed that whites were not susceptible to the disease. It was called "Nigger itch," or, where it was associated with immigrants, "Italian itch" or "Mexican bump." When smallpox broke out in New York City, police officers were sent to help enforce the vaccination of Italian and Irish immigrants in the tenements. And when smallpox arrived in Middlesboro, Kentucky, everyone in the black section of town who resisted vaccination was vaccinated at gunpoint. These campaigns did limit the spread of the disease, but all the risk of vaccination, which at that time could lead to

31

infection with tetanus and other diseases, was absorbed by the most vulnerable groups. The poor were enlisted in the protection of the privileged.

Debates over vaccination, then as now, are often cast as debates over the integrity of science, though they could just as easily be understood as conversations about power. The working-class people who resisted Britain's 1853 provision for free, mandatory vaccination were concerned, in part, with their own freedom. Faced with fines, imprisonment, and the seizure of their property if they did not vaccinate their infants, they sometimes compared their predicament to slavery.

Vaccination, like slavery, raises some pressing questions about one's rights to one's own body. But as the historian Nadja Durbach has noted, antivaccinators were often more interested in abolition as a metaphor for individual liberty than they were in the cause as a shared purpose. It was not in the recklessly selfless spirit of John Brown, who was hanged with his sons for their doomed effort to free slaves, that white workers resisted vaccination. "Antivaccinators were quick to draw on the political, emotive, or rhetorical value of the slave, or of the colonized African," Durbach writes of the movement in Britain. "They were quicker still to claim that the suffering of white English citizens took precedence over that of the oppressed elsewhere." Their primary concern, in other words, was with people like them.

In her history of that movement, Durbach returns often to the idea that vaccine resisters saw their bodies "not as potentially contagious and thus dangerous to the social body, but as highly vulnerable to contamination and violation." Their bodies were, of course, both contagious and vulnerable. But in a time and place where the bodies of the poor were seen as a liability to public

health, as dangerous to others, it fell to the poor to articulate their vulnerability.

If it was meaningful then for the poor to assert that
they were not purely dangerous, I suspect it might be just
as meaningful now for the rest of us to accept that we are
not purely vulnerable. The middle class may be "threatened," but we are still, just by virtue of having bodies,
dangerous. Even the little bodies of children, which our
time encourages us to imagine as absolutely vulnerable,
are dangerous in their ability to spread disease. Think
of the unvaccinated boy in San Diego, for instance, who
returned from a trip to Switzerland in 2008 with a case
of measles that infected his two siblings, five schoolmates, and four children in his doctor's waiting room.
Three of those children were infants too young to be
vaccinated, and one had to be hospitalized.

Unvaccinated children, a 2004 analysis of CDC data
reveals, are more likely to be white, to have an older
married mother with a college education, and to live in a
household with an income of $75,000 or more—like my
child. Unvaccinated children also tend to be clustered
in the same areas, raising the probability that they will
contract a disease that can then be passed, once it is in circulation, to undervaccinated children. Undervaccinated
children, meaning children who have received some but
not all of their recommended immunizations, are more
likely to be black, to have a younger unmarried mother,
to have moved across state lines, and to live in poverty.

"Vaccination works," my father explains, "by enlisting
a majority in the protection of a minority." He means the
minority of the population that is particularly vulnerable
to a given disease. The elderly, in the case of influenza.
Newborns, in the case of pertussis. Pregnant women, in
the case of rubella. But when relatively wealthy white

33

women vaccinate our children, we may also be participating in the protection of some poor black children whose single mothers have recently moved and have not, as a product of circumstance rather than choice, fully vaccinated them. This is a radical inversion of the historical application of vaccination, which was once just another form of bodily servitude extracted from the poor for the benefit of the privileged. There is some truth, now, to the idea that public health is not strictly *for* people like me, but it is *through us*, literally through our bodies, that certain public health measures are enacted.

¶ "We talked about germs in school," my son told me after one of his first days of preschool. The pronoun and the past tense made this a challenging sentence that had taken him several minutes of silence to formulate. He was holding a "germ" constructed of tangled and tortured pipe cleaners that looked not entirely unlike the electron microscope photos in the immunology textbooks I paged through while he was in school. "What did you learn?" I asked. "Germs are really, really tiny and really, really dirty," he explained with enthusiasm, happy to share his new knowledge. "Yes," I agreed, "that's why we have to wash your hands when we get to school in the morning, to wash off the germs so they don't get on anyone else." He nodded gravely, "Germs can make you sick. Make you cough."

The conversation ended there, in part because my two-year-old had, in the span of a few simple sentences, completely articulated my entire knowledge of infectious agents. It was a sobering moment. Sometime after this exchange, I looked up *germ* in a medical dictionary and was reminded that the word is used in two ways. A germ is an organism that causes disease, or it is a part of the body capable of building new tissue. We use the same word for something that brings illness and something that brings growth. The root of the word being, of course, *seed*.

We need germs. Without exposure to germs, we now know, a child's immune system is prone to dysfunction. In 1989, the immunologist David Strachan proposed that having older siblings, belonging to a large family, and living in an environment that was not overly sanitized might help protect children from developing asthma and allergies. This "hygiene hypothesis" suggested that it was possible to be too clean and too free of disease.

As the hygiene hypothesis took hold, scientists

searched for one particular childhood disease that might prevent allergies, but this thinking gave way to the understanding that the overall diversity of germs in our environment is probably more important. In 2004, the microbiologist Graham Rook proposed an "old friends" hypothesis, in which he suggested that a healthy immune system is not achieved through childhood diseases, which are relatively new, but through exposure to ancient pathogens that have been with us since our hunter-gatherer days. These "old friends" include parasites and worms as well as the bacteria that colonize our skin, lungs, nose, throat, and gut.

The hygiene hypothesis is still sometimes interpreted as a reason not to prevent infectious disease. "For all we know," as a friend remarked to me, "diseases like measles may be essential to our health." But the native peoples of the Americas lived for millennia without measles until it was introduced to this hemisphere relatively recently, with devastating results. And even if we eliminate measles through vaccination, as is theoretically possible, an abundance of germs remain. There are, for instance, about a million different viruses in a teaspoon of sea water. We may not muck around with other organisms as much as we should, but we have no dearth of germs available to us on Earth.

Vaccination of humans has made one single virus extinct—the variola virus that causes smallpox. But novel viruses are constantly inventing themselves, as viruses have a special talent for genetic variation. Of all the varieties of germs, viruses may be the most vexing. They are mysterious creatures, parasitic and vampiric by nature. They are not exactly inanimate, but viruses are not, strictly speaking, alive. They do not eat, do not grow, and generally do not live in the manner that other living things live. Viruses must enter and inhabit a living cell in order to reproduce, or to do much of anything. On their own, they are little more than minuscule bits of inert genetic material, so small that they cannot be seen by an ordinary microscope. Once inside another cell, viruses use that cell's body to make more of themselves. The metaphor of a factory is often used to describe how viruses work—they enter a cell and force its equipment to produce thousands more viruses. But viruses strike me as more supernatural than industrial—they are zombies, or body snatchers, or vampires.

A virus can, on occasion, infect an organism in a way that ensures the viral DNA will be passed on to that organism's offspring as part of their genetic code. A rather surprising amount of the human genome is made up of debris from ancient viral infections. Some of that genetic material does nothing, so far as we know, some can trigger cancer under certain conditions, and some has become essential to our survival. The cells that form the outer layer of the placenta for a human fetus bind to each other using a gene that originated, long ago, from a virus. Though many viruses cannot reproduce without us, we ourselves could not reproduce without what we have taken from them.

Our own adaptive immune system, the branch of our immune system that develops long-lasting immunity, is thought to have borrowed its essential technology from the DNA of a virus. Some of our white blood cells recombine their genetic material like random number generators, shuffling their sequenes to create an immense variety of cells capable of recognizing an immense variety of pathogens. This technology was viral technology before it was ours. Of humans and viruses, the science writer Carl Zimmer observes, "There is no us and them."

¶ The novel flu virus warnings issued by the CDC in my son's first year seemed to produce, more than anything else, a proliferation of antibacterial soap and hand sanitizer. Sanitizing wipes were stationed by the carts in grocery stores in addition to pumps of sanitizer at every check-out counter. Large pumps of sanitizer appeared at the entrance to security in the airport, in the post office, and at the circulation desk in my library. These sanitizers remained long after the threat of flu had abated.

I was reluctant to be routinely sanitized. My father, whose own hands were often cracked from repeated washing during his rounds in the hospital, had instilled in me a skepticism of anything that promised to kill germs. Not all germs should be put to death, he maintained. Killing germs, rather than washing them away, reminded him of the Crusades, when an abbot who was asked how to tell the faithful from the heretics replied, "Kill them all—God will know his own."

While hand sanitizers were killing indiscriminately, studies were finding the chemical triclosan in the urine of pregnant women, in the cord blood of newborn babies, and in the breast milk of nursing mothers. Triclosan, an antimicrobial agent used in toothpaste, mouthwash, deodorant, cleaning products, and laundry detergent, among other things, is also the active ingredient in nearly all antibacterial liquid soaps and many hand sanitizers.

What we know about triclosan is that at low concentrations it can prevent both "good" and "bad" microbes from reproducing, and at higher concentrations it can kill them. We know that it is in our wastewater, it is in our streams, and it is in our finished drinking water. It is in wild fish all over the world, it is in earthworms, and it is in the blood of bottlenose dolphins. What we do not know is exactly what this means for our ecosystem.

The upshot of quite a bit of research involving unfortunate mice, rats, and rabbits is that triclosan is probably not very toxic to humans. But the long-term effects of a lifetime of constant exposure are not yet known. Despite the protests of at least one large chemical company, the Food and Drug Administration nominated triclosan for further research at the National Toxicology Program in 2008. Scott Masten, the toxicologist I spoke with there, was rather dispassionate on the subject of triclosan. "I don't buy antibacterial soap," he allowed, when pressed, "not because I'm afraid of it, but because it doesn't have any benefit." A number of studies have found that washing with antibacterial soaps is actually no more effective at reducing bacteria than washing with regular soap and water. Triclosan is in soaps, Dr. Masten suggested, only because companies have found a market for antibacterial products that promise to kill rather than just clean.

I was interested, I explained to him, in thinking about how the risks posed by triclosan might compare to the risks posed by some of the components of vaccines. Our exposure to triclosan is nearly constant, and it can even be found in the urine of people who do not use any products that contain it. In comparison, our exposure to traces of other chemicals through vaccination is limited to a couple dozen instances. But I did not want to make the mistake of exaggerating the dangers associated with triclosan, I told Dr. Masten, in pursuit of this idea. "Relative risk problems are hard to communicate," he agreed. The health risks triclosan poses for humans are probably low, but any degree of risk, he reminded me, should be unacceptable in a product that does not do any good.

Fears of vaccines do not seem easily quieted by an abundance of expert risk-benefit analyses assuring us that the good they do is far greater than the harm. Serious side effects from vaccination are rare. But it is difficult to quantify exactly how rare, in part because many of the complications associated with vaccines are also caused by the natural infections those vaccines are designed to prevent. Natural infections of measles, mumps, chicken pox, and influenza can all cause encephalitis, a swelling of the brain. We do not know what the base rate of encephalitis would be in a population with no disease and no vaccination against disease. But we do know that 1 in about every 1,000 cases of measles leads to encephalitis, and that encephalitis has been reported after vaccination in about 1 out of every 3 million doses of the MMR (measles-mumps-rubella) vaccine. This incidence is so rare that researchers have been unable to definitely determine whether or not encephalitis is caused by the vaccine.

A comprehensive report on vaccine "adverse events" was released in 2011 by a committee of eighteen medical experts who reviewed 12,000 studies of vaccination for the Institute of Medicine. They found convincing evidence that the MMR vaccine can, very rarely, cause a condition called measles inclusion body encephalitis in people with compromised immune systems. The MMR can also cause fever-induced seizures that are usually mild and result in no long-term harm. The chicken pox vaccine can cause chicken pox, particularly in people with weakened immune systems. And six different vaccines can cause an anaphylactic allergic reaction in people with severe allergies. The injection of any type of vaccine can produce fainting and muscle pain caused not by the vaccine, but by the act of injection itself.

What vaccines do not cause, the report explained, is significantly harder to establish than what they do cause. While a substantial amount of evidence is acceptable as proof that an event does and can happen, there is never enough evidence to prove that an event cannot happen. Even so, the evidence reviewed by the committee "favors rejection" of the theory that the MMR vaccine causes autism. This report was released shortly after a national survey revealed that a quarter of the parents who responded believed that vaccines cause autism. And over half of the parents expressed concern about serious side effects from vaccines.

"Perceptions of risk—the intuitive judgments that people make about the hazards of their world," the historian Michael Willrich observes, "can be stubbornly resistant to the evidence of experts." We do not tend to be afraid of the things that are most likely to harm us. We drive around in cars, a lot. We drink alcohol, we ride bicycles, we sit too much. And we harbor anxiety about things that, statistically speaking, pose us little danger. We fear sharks, while mosquitoes are, in terms of sheer numbers of lives lost, probably the most dangerous creature on earth.

"Do people know which risks lead to many deaths and which risks lead to few?" the legal scholar Cass Sunstein asks. "They do not. In fact, they make huge blunders." Sunstein draws this observation from the work of Paul Slovic, author of *The Perception of Risk*. In a study that invited people to compare various causes of death, Slovic found that people tended to believe that accidents cause more deaths than disease and that homicide causes more deaths than suicide, when the opposite is true in both cases. In another study, people significantly overestimated the fatality rates of highly publicized or dramatic dangers like cancer or tornadoes.

One could interpret this, as Sunstein does, to mean that most people are just wrong about risk. But risk perception may not be about quantifiable risk so much as it is about immeasurable fear. Our fears are informed by history and economics, by social power and stigma, by myths and nightmares. And as with other strongly held beliefs, our fears are dear to us. When we encounter information that contradicts our beliefs, as Slovic found in one of his studies, we tend to doubt the information, not ourselves.

Bicycles, the *New York Times* reports, "are involved in more accidents than any other consumer product, but beds rank a close second." This does not alarm me, though I am a frequent user of both beds and bicycles. I carry my son on the back of my bicycle and allow him to sleep in my bed, despite public service posters of a baby sleeping with a butcher knife that warn me, "Your baby sleeping with you can be just as dangerous." The disregard for statistical risk that researchers observe in people like me may be at least partly due to an unwillingness to live lives dictated by danger. We sleep with our babies because the benefits, as we see them, outweigh the risks. The birth of my son, which posed a greater risk to my health than I anticipated when I became pregnant, gave me a new appreciation for the idea that there are some risks worth taking. "Having children," a friend with grown children reminds me, "is the greatest risk you can take."

"Perhaps what matters," Sunstein muses, "is not whether people are right on the facts, but whether they are frightened." And people do seem to be frightened. We are locking our doors and pulling our children out of public school and buying guns and ritually sanitizing our hands to allay a wide range of fears, most of which are essentially fears of other people. All the while we are also, in our way, reckless. We get *intoxicated*, from the Latin "to poison," for fun. This contradiction leads Sunstein to worry that regulatory laws based on the priorities of the general public may be prone to a pattern of "paranoia and neglect." Too much attention may be spent on minimal risks, while too little is paid to pressing threats.

Paranoia, the theorist Eve Sedgwick observes, tends to be contagious. She calls it a "strong theory," meaning a wide-ranging, reductive theory that displaces other ways of thinking. And paranoia very frequently passes for intelligence. As Sedgwick observes, "to theorize out of anything *but* a paranoid critical stance has come to seem naïve, pious, or complaisant." She does not believe that paranoid thinking is necessarily delusional or wrong, but only that there is value to approaches that are less rooted in suspicion. "Paranoia," Sedgwick writes, "knows some things well and others poorly."

Intuitive toxicology is the term that Slovic uses for the way most people assess the risk of chemicals. His research reveals that this approach is distinct from the methods used by toxicologists, and that it tends to produce different results. For toxicologists, "the dose makes the poison." Any substance can be toxic in excess. Water, for instance, is lethal to humans in very high doses, and overhydration killed a runner in the 2002 Boston Marathon. But most people prefer to think of substances as either safe or dangerous, regardless of the dose. And we extend this thinking to exposure, in that we regard any exposure to chemicals, no matter how brief or limited, as harmful.

In exploring this thinking, Slovic suggests that people

who are not toxicologists may apply a "law of contagion" to toxicity. Just as brief exposure to a microscopic virus can result in lifelong disease, we assume that exposure to any amount of a harmful chemical will permanently contaminate our bodies. "Being contaminated," Slovic observes, "clearly has an all-or-none quality to it—like being alive or pregnant."

Fear of contamination rests on the belief, widespread in our culture as in others, that something can impart its essence to us on contact. We are forever polluted, as we see it, by contact with a pollutant. And the pollutants we have come to fear most are the products of our own hands. Though toxicologists tend to disagree with this, many people regard natural chemicals as inherently less harmful than man-made chemicals. We seem to believe, against all evidence, that nature is entirely benevolent.

¶ One of the appeals of alternative medicine is that it offers not just an alternative philosophy or an alternative treatment but also an alternative language. If we feel polluted, we are offered a "cleanse." If we feel inadequate, lacking, we are offered a "supplement." If we fear toxins, we are offered "detoxification." If we fear that we are rusting with age, physically oxidizing, we are reassured with "antioxidants." These are metaphors that address our base anxieties. And what the language of alternative medicine understands is that when we feel bad we want something unambiguously good.

Most of the pharmaceuticals available to us are at least as bad as they are good. My father has the habit of saying, "There are very few perfect therapies in medicine." True as it may be, the idea that our medicine is as flawed as we are is not comforting. And when comfort is what we want, one of the most powerful tonics alternative medicine offers is the word *natural*. This word implies a medicine untroubled by human limitations, contrived wholly by nature or God or perhaps intelligent design. What *natural* has come to mean to us in the context of medicine is *pure* and *safe* and *benign*. But the use of *natural* as a synonym for *good* is almost certainly a product of our profound alienation from the natural world.

"Obviously," the naturalist Wendell Berry writes, "the more artificial a human environment becomes, the more the word 'natural' becomes a term of value." If, he argues, "we see the human and the natural economies as necessarily opposite or opposed, we subscribe to the very opposition that threatens to destroy them both. The wild and the domestic now often seem isolated values, estranged from one another. And yet these are not exclusive polarities like good and evil. There can be continuity between them, and there must be."

Allowing children to develop immunity to contagious diseases "naturally," without vaccination, is appealing to some of us. Much of that appeal depends on the belief that vaccines are inherently unnatural. But vaccines are of that liminal place between humans and nature— a mowed field, Berry might suggest, edged by woods. Vaccination is a kind of domestication of a wild thing, in that it involves our ability to harness a virus and break it like a horse, but its action depends on the natural response of the body to the effects of that once-wild thing.

The antibodies that generate immunity following vaccination are manufactured in the human body, not in factories. "In the pharmaceutical world," the writer Jane Smith observes, "the great division is between biologicals and chemicals—drugs that are made from living substances and drugs that are made from chemical compounds." Using ingredients sourced from organisms, once living or still alive, vaccines invite the immune system to produce its own protection. The live viruses in vaccines are weakened, sometimes by having been passed through the bodies of animals, so that they cannot infect a healthy person. The most unnatural aspect of vaccination is that it does not, when all goes well, introduce disease or produce illness.

Infectious disease is one of the primary mechanisms of natural immunity. Whether we are sick or healthy, disease is always passing through our bodies. "Probably we're diseased all the time," as one biologist puts it, "but we're hardly ill." It is only when disease manifests as illness that we see it as unnatural, in the "contrary to the ordinary course of nature" sense of the word. When a child's fingers blacken on his hand from Hib disease, when tetanus locks a child's jaw and stiffens her body, when a baby barks for breath from pertussis, when a child's legs are twisted and shrunken with polio—then disease does not seem natural.

Before Christopher Columbus landed in the Bahamas, the epidemic diseases of Europe and Asia did not exist in the Americas. There was no smallpox, no hepatitis, no measles, no influenza. The bacteria that cause diphtheria, tuberculosis, cholera, typhus, and scarlet fever were all unknown in this hemisphere. "The first recorded epidemic, perhaps due to swine flu, was in 1493," Charles Mann writes in his book *1493*. From that year onward, earthworms and honeybees imported by Europeans would forever change the ecology of the Americas, cattle and apple trees would transform its landscape, and novel diseases would decimate its people. Within the next two hundred years, three-quarters or more of the native population of the Americas would die of disease. Considering this course of events "natural" favors the perspective of the people who subsequently colonized the land, but it fails to satisfy the "not made or caused by humankind" definition of the term. While the ecosystem of the Americas can never be restored to its pre-Columbian state, our efforts to limit epidemic diseases through vaccination may be one small measure of habitat restoration.

"The history of the recent centuries has its black passages—the slaughter of the buffalo on the western plains, the massacre of the shorebirds by the market gunners, the near-extermination of the egrets for their plumage," Rachel Carson wrote in *Silent Spring*. She was writing in the late fifties, at a moment of acute atomic awareness, and the next of these black passages would be, she warned, a "new kind of fallout." The pesticides and herbicides of postwar industry, some of them originally developed for war, were being sprayed from airplanes over acres of fields and forests. One of these, DDT, was making its way into groundwater, accumulating in fish, and killing birds. Over fifty years later, DDT persists in the bodies of fish and birds all over the world, as well as in the milk of nursing mothers.

The publication of *Silent Spring* in 1962 led to the creation of the Environmental Protection Agency and a ban on the production of DDT in the United States. The book popularized the idea that human health depends on the health of the ecosystem as a whole, but Carson did not use the word *ecosystem*. She preferred the metaphor of an "intricate web of life," in which a disturbance anywhere on the web sends tremors across the entire web. "*Silent Spring*," Carson's biographer Linda Lear writes, "proved that our bodies are not boundaries."

Our bodies are not boundaries, but DDT is not exactly what Carson feared it was. DDT, she warned, was a widespread cause of cancer. This hypothesis was not supported by the decades of research on DDT that followed the publication of *Silent Spring*. Numerous studies on factory and farm workers with high DDT exposure failed to find an association between DDT and cancer. And studies of specific cancers found no evidence that DDT increased the incidence of breast cancer, lung cancer, testicular cancer, liver cancer, or prostate cancer. I mention this to my father, an oncologist, and he recalls the DDT sprayed all over his town from trucks when he was young. He and his siblings were kept inside during the spraying, but they ran out to play as soon as the trucks had passed, when the leaves of trees were still dripping DDT and the smell of the chemical was in the air. It does not bother him that Carson may have overstated some of the dangers of DDT, and that she got some things wrong, because, as he says, "she got the job done." She woke us up.

"Few books have done more to change the world," the journalist Tina Rosenberg acknowledges. "DDT killed bald eagles because of its persistence in the environment," she writes. "*Silent Spring* is now killing African children because of its persistence in the public mind." The blame for this may belong more to us, the inheritors of *Silent Spring*, than to the book, but either way malaria has re-surged in some countries where DDT is no longer used against mosquitoes. One African child in twenty now dies from malaria, and more are left brain damaged by the disease. Ineffective treatments, toxic prophylactics, and environmentally damaging insecticides all remain in use because there is no viable vaccine against malaria.

For now, DDT is, unfortunately, one of the more eff-ective means of controlling malaria in some places. App-lied to the interior walls of homes once a year, DDT has nearly eliminated malaria in parts of South Africa. Compared to spraying DDT across millions of acres from airplanes, as was done in the United States, the en-vironmental impact of this application is relatively small. But DDT remains an imperfect solution. Few chemical companies produce it, donors are unwilling to finance it, and many countries are reluctant to use a chemical that is banned elsewhere. "Probably the worst thing that ever happened to malaria in poor nations," Rosenberg writes, "was its eradication in rich ones."

Colonization and the slave trade brought malaria to the Americas, where it was once common as far north as Boston. Malaria never had quite as strong a hold in this country as it has in Africa, but it was difficult to erad-icate here nonetheless. Beginning around the 1920s, thousands of miles of ditches were dug, swamps were drained, window screens were installed, and tons of an arsenic-based insecticide were spread. This was all to destroy breeding grounds and repel the mosquitoes that spread malaria. In a final push, DDT was applied to the walls of millions of homes, insecticides were sprayed from airplanes, and malaria was eliminated from the United States by 1949. Among other advantages, this contributed to the growth of our economy. Matthew Bonds, an economist at Harvard Medical School, compares the global effects of disease to widespread crime or government corruption. "Infectious diseases," he says, "systematically steal human resources."

"Such a catalog of illnesses!" Carson complained to a friend when an eye inflammation left her unable to read her own writing. Her work on *Silent Spring* had already been slowed by an ulcer, pneumonia, a staph infection, and two tumors. She kept this cancer, which would kill her shortly after the publication of *Silent Spring*, a secret. She did not want her work to appear to be driven by anything other than scientific evidence. And so her personal struggle with cancer was told only through dwindling numbers of bald eagles, through eggs that did not hatch, and through the robins that lay dead on the lawns of suburbia.

Even as Carson proposed that DDT could cause cancer, she recognized its utility for disease prevention. "No responsible person," she wrote, "contends that insect-borne disease should be ignored." Chemicals should be used in response to real threats, she suggested, rather than "mythical situations." She advocated for the informed, judicious use of chemicals, not the neglect of African children. But the enduring power of her book owes less to its nuances than to its capacity to induce horror.

Silent Spring begins with a "Fable for Tomorrow" in which Carson imagines an idyllic landscape of oaks, ferns, and wildflowers that is rapidly transformed into an apocalyptic wasteland where birds no longer sing. In the pages that follow, workers who have been picking oranges fall violently ill, a housewife who hates spiders develops leukemia, and a boy who runs to greet his father, just back from spraying the potato fields, dies that night from pesticide poisoning. It is a horror story in which man's creation, his monster, turns against him. Like Dracula, this monster moves through the air as mist and lies dormant in the soil. And like the plot of *Dracula*, the drama of *Silent Spring* depends on emblematic oppositions—good and evil, human and inhuman, natural and unnatural, ancient and modern. The monster in *Dracula* has ancient origins, but in *Silent Spring* evil takes the form of modern life.

¶ Triclosan is destroying our environment and slowly poisoning us all, I determined shortly after I began reading about its toxicity. Or, triclosan is harmless to humans and not a serious threat to the environment. Uncertain how to interpret the data, I called the author of one of the studies I had read, an FDA researcher with a kindly voice. I explained my problem and he said that he would like to help me, but he was not supposed to talk to the press. It had not occurred to me that I was the press, though I was writing an article for *Harper's* magazine at the time.

Frustrated, I hung up the phone and fell asleep with my face on a pile of articles about herd immunity. I woke to find that a fragment of print had been transferred to my cheek. It spelled "munity," from the Latin *munis* for service or duty. "Munity is what you are really writing about," a colleague would say to me months later, "not immunity." This struck me as true, though I was writing about both.

As I rode my bicycle to my son's preschool after failing to determine how good or bad triclosan might be, it began to rain. I ran one block from the school to the public library through the rain, carrying my son, who was laughing. Inside, he darted through the stacks selecting picture books at random, while the question of whether or not I was the press continued to bother me. I understood it as a broader question of belonging. In my mind, I do not belong to the press even if my writing is published by the press. And if the opposite of the press is a poet, then I am both.

My son returned with a book about a baby alien who gets lost on Earth where nobody speaks her language, a book about a bat who lives with a family of birds who do not hang upside down like she does, and a book about a monkey who is teased for walking on two legs instead of four. The wordplay in *Gakky Two-Feet* was very funny to my son, but he did not understand the central conflict. Why, he wondered, does it bother the other monkeys when Gakky walks on two feet? "They feel threatened by his difference," I said. "What does *threatened* mean?" he asked.

It took me some time to define *threatened* because I was looking back through the books. Belonging and not belonging is a common theme of children's books, and maybe of childhood itself, but I was surprised that all these books were about the same thing. They were all about the problem of "us" and "them." The bat does not really belong with the birds even though she lives with the birds, and the alien is not at home on Earth. In the end, the bat is reunited with her bat mother and the alien is rescued by her alien parents, but some questions remain. "How can we be so different and feel so much alike?" one of the birds asks the bat. "And how can we feel so different and be so much alike?" another bird wonders.

Bats and birds may be of different biological classes, but they are both, as any child can see, flying things. *Stellaluna*, the book about the bat, allows for some confusion of categories, some disruption of boundaries. But "us" and "them" thinking insists on one belonging firmly to one category or another—it does not make room for ambiguous identities or outsider insiders. It does not allow for bat-bird alliances or resident aliens or monkeys who are in the process of evolving. And so the opposition between "us" and "them" becomes, as Wendell Berry warns, "the very opposition that threatens to destroy them both."

"I know you're on my side," an immunologist once re-marked to me as we discussed the politics of vaccination. I did not agree with him, but only because I was uncomfortable with both sides, as I had seen them delineated. The debate over vaccination tends to be described with what the philosopher of science Donna Haraway would call "troubling dualisms." These dualisms pit science against nature, public against private, truth against imagination, self against other, thought against emotion, and man against woman.

The metaphor of a "war" between mothers and doctors is sometimes used for conflicts over vaccination. Depending on who is employing the metaphor, the warring parties may be characterized as ignorant mothers and educated doctors, or intuitive mothers and intellectual doctors, or caring mothers and heartless doctors, or irrational mothers and rational doctors—sexist stereotypes abound.

Rather than imagine a war in which we are ultimately fighting against ourselves, perhaps we can accept a world in which we are all irrational rationalists. We are bound, in this world, to both nature and technology. We are all "cyborgs, hybrids, mosaics, chimeras," as Haraway suggests in her feminist provocation "A Cyborg Manifesto." She envisions a cyborg world "in which people are not afraid of their joint kinship with animals and machines, not afraid of permanently partial identities and contradictory standpoints."

All of us who have been vaccinated are cyborgs, the cyborg scholar Chris Hables Gray suggests. Our bodies have been programmed to respond to disease, and modified by technologically altered viruses. As a cyborg and a nursing mother, I join my modified body to a breast pump, a modern mechanism, to provide my child with the most primitive food. On my bicycle, I am part human and part machine, a collaboration that exposes me to injury. Our technology both extends and endangers us. Good or bad, it is part of us, and this is no more unnatural than it is natural.

When a friend asked, years ago, if my son's birth was a "natural" birth, I was tempted to say that it was an animal birth. While his head was crowning, I was trying to use my own hands to pull apart my flesh and bring him out of my body. Or so I have been told, but I do not remember any intention to tear myself open—all I remember is the urgency of the moment. I was both human and animal then. Or I was neither, as I am now. "We have never been human," Haraway suggests. And perhaps we have never been modern, either.

¶ Vaccination is a precursor to modern medicine, not the product of it. Its roots are in folk medicine, and its first practitioners were farmers. Milkmaids in eighteenth-century England had faces unblemished by smallpox. Nobody knew why, but anyone could see it was true. Nearly everyone in England at that time got smallpox and many of those who survived bore the scars of the disease on their faces. Folk knowledge held that if a milkmaid milked a cow blistered with cowpox and developed some blisters on her hands, she would not contract smallpox even while nursing victims of an epidemic.

By the end of the century, just as the waterwheels of the industrial revolution were beginning to turn the spindles in cotton mills, physicians were noting the effects of cowpox on milkmaids and anyone who milked cows. During a smallpox epidemic in 1774, a farmer who had himself already been infected with cowpox used a darning needle to drive pus from a cow into the arms of his wife and two small boys. The farmer's neighbors were horrified. His wife's arm became red and swollen and she fell ill before recovering fully, but the boys had mild reactions. They were exposed to smallpox many times over the course of their long lives, occasionally for the purpose of demonstrating their immunity, without ever contracting the disease.

Twenty years later, the country doctor Edward Jenner extracted pus from a blister on the hand of a milkmaid and scraped it into the arm of an eight-year-old boy. The boy got a fever but did not become ill. Jenner then exposed the boy to smallpox, which did not infect him. Emboldened, Jenner continued his experiment on dozens of other people, including his own infant son. Before long, the procedure would be known by Jenner's term for cowpox, *variolae vaccinae*, from the Latin *vacca* for cow, the beast that would forever leave its mark on vaccination.

Jenner had the evidence to suggest that vaccination worked, but he did not know why it worked. His innovation was based entirely on observation, not on theory. This was a century before the first virus would be identified, and long before the cause of smallpox would be understood. Surgeons did not yet have anesthesia, nor did they know to sterilize their equipment. Nearly a century would pass before germ theory would be validated, and well over a century would pass before penicillin would be extracted from a fungus.

The basic mechanism behind vaccination was not new even when an intrepid dairy farmer used a darning needle to vaccinate his children. At that point, variolation, the practice of purposefully infecting a person with a mild case of smallpox in order to prevent more serious illness, was still somewhat novel in England but had been practiced in China and India for hundreds of years. Variolation would ultimately be brought to America from Africa. The procedure was explained to the Puritan minister Cotton Mather by his Libyan slave Onesimus. When Mather asked him if he had ever had smallpox, Onesimus replied, "Yes and no." What he meant is that he had been inoculated with smallpox as a child, like many other slaves born in Africa.

Mather, who had lost a wife and three children to measles, convinced a local doctor to inoculate two slaves and the doctor's own young son when an epidemic of smallpox spread through Boston in 1721. After these first three patients recovered, the doctor went on to inoculate several hundred people, whose rate of survival would prove much better than that of those who had not been inoculated. Mather, the author of an account of the Salem witch trials that was considered overzealous even in his time, began preaching that variolation was a gift from God, a sentiment so unpopular that a firebomb was thrown through his window. The accompanying message read, "Cotton Mather, you dog. Damn you! I'll inoculate you with this with a pox to you."

Variolation was introduced to England at about the same time by Mary Wortley Montagu, who had her six-year-old son and her two-year-old daughter inoculated after observing the practice in Turkey. Montagu, the wife of a British ambassador, had lost her brother to smallpox and her own face was badly scarred from the disease. The princess of Wales, having also survived smallpox, arranged for variolation to be tested on prisoners condemned to die. The prisoners lived, immune to smallpox, and were freed for their trouble. The princess, who would later become queen when her husband became George II, inoculated her seven children.

By the time Voltaire published his *Letters Concerning the English Nation* in 1733, variolation was widely practiced in England, though still feared in France. Himself a survivor of a serious case of smallpox, Voltaire suggested that if the French had adopted the practice as readily as the English, "twenty thousand persons whom the smallpox swept away at Paris in 1723 would have been alive at this time."

When Voltaire wrote "On Inoculation," the primary meaning of the English word *inoculate* was still to set a bud or scion, as apples are cultivated by grafting a stem from one tree onto the roots of another. There were many methods of inoculation, including the snuffing of dried and ground scabs up the nose or the sewing of an infected thread through the webbing between the thumb and finger, but in England it was often practiced by making a slit or flap in the skin into which infectious material was placed, like the slit in the bark of a tree that receives the young stem grafted to it. When the word *inoculate* was first used to describe variolation, it was a metaphor for grafting a disease, which would bear its own fruit, to the rootstock of the body.

¶ Our understanding of immunity remains remarkably dependent on metaphor, even at the most technical level. Immunologists describe the activities of our cells with terms like interpretation and communication, imbuing them with essentially human characteristics. Three immunologists on a road trip in 1984 became excited about the possibility that the cells of our bodies might, like the humans they compose, use a system of signs and symbols—a kind of language—in their communication with each other. After traveling for seventeen hours in a VW bus with a ripe wheel of Taleggio cheese and an Italian edition of Umberto Eco's *A Theory of Semiotics*, they determined, through some rough translations performed by the Italian among them, that a better understanding of semiotics, the study of how signs and symbols are used and interpreted, might enhance their work in immunology.

When I learned of the resulting conference on "immunosemiotics," I was excited by the possibility that it was devoted to the discussion of metaphor, a semiotic device. I thought I had found a group of immunologists interested in dissecting their own metaphors. To my disappointment, the conference papers revealed that they were much more concerned with the question of how our bodies, not our minds, interpret symbols. But as the immunologist Franco Celada proposed in a paper titled "Does the Human Mind Use a Logic of Signs Developed by Lymphocytes 10^8 Years Ago?" our minds may have learned the ability to interpret from our bodies.

"Immunologists are forced to use unusual expressions in order to describe their observations," the semiotician Thure von Uexküll observed at the conference. "Expressions like 'memory,' 'recognition,' 'interpretation,' 'individuality,' 'reading,' 'inner picture,' 'self,' 'nonself,'" he maintained, were unknown in physics or chemistry. "Atoms and molecules have no self, memory, individuality, or inner pictures," he said. "They are not able to read, to recognise or to interpret anything and cannot be killed either." Some of the other semioticians at that conference, most notably Umberto Eco, would question whether the cells of the body were literally engaged in acts of interpretation, but the immunologists seemed less skeptical.

When the anthropologist Emily Martin asked an array of scientists to discuss descriptions of the immune system that depended on the metaphor of a body at war, some of them rejected the idea that this was a metaphor. It was, they insisted, "how it is." One scientist disliked the war metaphor, but only because he objected to the way war was being waged at that moment. In her study of how we think about immunity, which was conducted during the first Iraq war, Martin found that metaphors of military defense permeate our imagination of the immune system.

"Popular publications," Martin observes, "depict the body as the scene of total war between ruthless invaders and determined defenders." Our understanding of disease as something that we "fight" invites an array of military metaphors for the immune system. In illustrated books and magazine articles, the body employs some cells as "infantry" and others as the "armored unit," and these troops deploy "mines" to explode bacteria, while the immune response itself "detonates like a bomb."

But this war imagery does not reflect the full diversity of thinking Martin discovered in her interviews. Alternative medicine practitioners, as a group, consistently refused to use war metaphors in their descriptions of the immune system. Most other people, scientists and nonscientists alike, tended to gravitate toward militaristic terms, but many were able to suggest different metaphors and some explicitly resisted military metaphors. "My visualization would be much more like a piece of almost tides or something … the forces, you know, the ebbs and flows," a lawyer remarked, clarifying that by forces she meant "imbalance and balance." A number of other people, including scientists, echoed this idea of a body striving for balance and harmony, rather than engaging in armed conflict. The inventive metaphors with which they imagined the immune system ranged from a symphony to the solar system to a perpetual motion machine to the vigilance of a mother.

The term *immune system* was used for the first time in 1967 by Niels Jerne, an immunologist who was trying to reconcile two factions of immunology—those who believed that immunity depended largely on antibodies and those who believed it depended more on specialized cells. Jerne used the word *system* to unite all the cells and antibodies and organs involved in immunity into one comprehensive whole. This idea that immunity is the product of a complex system of interdependent parts acting in concert is relatively new to science.

Even so, what we know of this system is staggering. It begins at the skin, a barrier capable of synthesizing biochemicals that inhibit the growth of certain bacteria and containing, in its deeper layers, cells that can induce inflammation and ingest pathogens. Then there are the membranes of the digestive, respiratory, and urogenital systems with their pathogen-ensnaring mucous and their pathogen-expelling cilia and their high concentration of cells equipped to produce the antibodies responsible for lasting immunity. Beyond those barriers, the circulatory system transports pathogens in the blood to the spleen, where the blood is filtered and antibodies are generated, and the lymphatic system flushes pathogens from body tissues to the lymph nodes, where the same process ensues—pathogens are surrounded by an assortment of cells that ingest them, eliminate them, and remember them for a more efficient response in the future.

Deep in the body, the bone marrow and the thymus generate a dizzying array of cells specialized for immunity. These include cells that can destroy infected cells, cells that swallow pathogens and then display pieces of them for other cells to see, cells that monitor other cells for signs of cancer or infection, cells that make antibodies, and cells that carry antibodies. All of these cells, falling into an intricate arrangement of types and subtypes, interact in a series of baroque dances, their communication depending in part on the action of free-floating molecules. Chemical signals travel through the blood from sites of injury or infection, activated cells release substances to trigger inflammation, and helpful molecules poke holes in the membranes of microbes to deflate them.

Infants have all the components of this system at birth. There are certain things the infant immune system does not do well—it has trouble penetrating the sticky coating of the Hib bacteria, for example. But the immune system of a full-term infant is not incomplete or undeveloped. It is what immunologists call "naive." It has not yet had the opportunity to produce antibodies in response to infection. Infants are born with some antibodies from their mothers already circulating in their systems, and breast milk supplies them with more antibodies, but this "passive immunity" fades as an infant grows, no matter how long it is breast-fed. A vaccine tutors the infant immune system, making it capable of remembering pathogens it has not yet seen. With or without vaccination, the first years of a child's life are a time of rapid education on immunity—all the runny noses and fevers of those years are the symptoms of a system learning the microbial lexicon.

When I asked for help understanding the basic mechanics of immunity, a professor of immunology gave me a two-hour explanation of the immune system in a coffee shop. He never once, in those two hours, used a military metaphor to describe the workings of the body. His metaphors tended to be gastronomic or educational—cells "ate" or "digested" pathogens and "instructed" other cells. When he spoke of something being killed or destroyed, he was referring to literal death or destruction. The scientific term for a type of white blood cell capable of destroying other cells, he told me, is *natural killer*.

Later, I attended a series of lectures by the same professor. While I was learning the distinction between innate immunity and adaptive immunity and trying desperately to keep track of a proliferation of acronyms —NLRs and PAMPs and APCs—I would note that the cells of the immune system lead lives in which they kiss, are naive, eat, purge, express, get turned on, are instructed, make presentations, mature, and have memories. "They sound like my students," a friend of mine, a poetry professor, would observe.

If a narrative of any kind emerged from those lectures, it was the drama of the interaction between our immune system and the pathogens with which it co-evolved. This drama was sometimes characterized as an ongoing battle, but not the kind that involves Apache helicopters and unmanned drones—this was clearly a battle of the wits. "And then the viruses got even smarter," my professor would say, "and did something ingenious—they used our own strategies against us." In his telling, our bodies and the viruses were two competing intelligences locked in a mortal game of chess.

¶ I walk the edge of a large cemetery whenever I walk north along Lake Michigan, which is nearly every day when the weather is warm. One high summer morning when my son was clamoring to get out of his stroller, I turned through the iron gate of the cemetery so that he could run on its paths under the shade of its trees. "Hi," he called out brightly, waving into space as we entered the empty cemetery. "Hi," he kept saying as he toddled down the path, pausing to smile and wave at nothing. I had only ever heard him say "hi" to people, so I knelt down to catch his sight line and saw that he was staring at the doors of a tomb. "What's that?" he asked, and I chilled. But now he was careening down the path and I followed him, pausing in front of a granite obelisk that caught my eye because it was inscribed with the first name WILLIE in large letters where the family name appeared on other stones. Willie had died in 1888, at the age of eight.

"Hi," my son was saying again, somewhat insistently, a few feet away, "hi!" He was standing in front of a marble statue of a little boy. The boy had the full cheeks of a baby and his marble eyes stared gravely into the middle distance. An eroded stone at my feet revealed that his name was Josie and he had died in 1891 at nine years old. As my son reached out his hand toward the boy I caught his wrist, in a rising panic, saying, "No, don't touch that!" I still cannot say exactly what scared me in that moment. Did I worry that my son would catch death if he touched the marble boy?

After leaving the cemetery I remarked to my father that I had noticed the graves of five-year-olds and ten-year-olds and a number of teenagers, but that I was surprised not to have seen, in one of the oldest cemeteries in Chicago, the graves of any babies. This, my father reminded me, was probably because infants died in such large numbers during the nineteenth century that they were not routinely buried in marked graves. Later, I would learn that one out of every ten children born in 1900 died before their first birthdays. I would read this in a report on vaccine side effects, which concluded its brief historical overview of child mortality with the observation that now "children are expected to survive to adulthood."

The first night my son slept farther than an arm's length from me, I fell asleep with the baby monitor pressed painfully against my ear. When the monitor ran out of batteries and began to beep I woke in alarm, but my son continued to sleep. His crib was no more than twelve feet from my bed, with an open door between us, and I could hear him crying quite well without a monitor, but I wanted to hear him breathing. I understood that this was an absurd indulgence but it was one I could not resist. The monitor, when it was turned up loudly enough for me to imagine I could hear breathing, produced a thick static that hosted a range of otherworldly sounds. I heard low muttering and whispering, clicks and bumps and sometimes crashes that were, when I rushed to see, nothing. Occasionally the monitor picked up phone conversations and I heard voices clearly for a few moments. I often woke in the night to crying that disappeared as soon as I was fully awake, and this happened, I began to notice, at the same time every night, just as a jet plane came in low over the lake to land at O'Hare. My sleeping mind, I realized, was choosing the frequencies it was listening for and manufacturing the crying of a baby out of the combination of the whine of the jet plane's engines and the static of the baby monitor. *Psycho acoustics*, a musician friend of mine once called this phenomenon.

I stopped using the baby monitor finally because I had to admit to myself that I did not know what I was listening for. But I continued to listen. One evening shortly after my son turned two, I heard a strange sound from his room just as I was getting into bed. I was no longer finding crying in the whine of jet planes, but I still sometimes woke with a start from a dream of crying. This sound I heard could have been a dog in the courtyard or it could have been a chair scraping the floor upstairs. I was only certain that I had really heard it because I heard it once more, and then there was a long silence. I walked to my son's door and listened. He was asleep, I was certain.

It was dark and quiet in his room, as usual, but he was sitting up in bed. Tears were running down his face and his mouth was wide open, gasping silently. I grabbed him, heard a thin whine of breath pulling through his throat, and laid him over my knees in an attempt at the Heimlich maneuver. This had worked for me in the past, but it produced nothing this time and only further alarmed my boy, whose body was quivering with fear. My husband, out of bed now, swept the back of his throat, found nothing, and carried him directly out the door for the hospital.

When I ran into the emergency room ten minutes later with my son's mouth next to my ear, saying, "He's having trouble breathing!" the triage nurse was unimpressed. "It's probably stridor," she said to her computer screen. Stridor, I would learn, is the high-pitched wheezing sound that indicates an obstructed airway. But as the nurse could see, my son's color was good and his breathing was better, having improved, to my surprise, after we took him out into the cold night air. By the time the doctor arrived, my son was coughing the strange, barking cough I had heard from his room. "I'd know that cough anywhere," the doctor said cheerfully. "I don't even need to look at him to make this diagnosis." It was *croup*, a swelling of the throat caused by a viral infection. Croup can be mild or severe, depending on the size of a child's airway, and it produces a distinctive cough that can lead to stridor and difficulty breathing. Beyond being what the doctor termed "moderately severe," this was a typical case of croup, having appeared at night in a toddler who seemed well when he was put to bed. Cold air, a traditional treatment for croup, had eased the swelling and reduced his stridor on the way to the hospital.

I had been up unusually late that night, I told the doctor, but if I had not already been awake I might not have heard those two little barking coughs before the stridor set in, and I might not have discovered that my son could not breathe. I left the next part unstated, my certainty that this could have killed him, but the doctor understood. No, he explained, this could be a frightening illness, but my son was getting enough air to live. He might have been very uncomfortable and very scared without me, but he would not have died before morning.

A few days later, I ran into a mother whose child often played with mine at the park field house when it was too cold to play outside. She was a young woman, usually tireless, who today looked weary. Her daughter had croup and had been coughing all night for days, she told me, and another boy we knew from the field house had been sick for over a week. Most of the small children who played in that big gym, I would learn, had caught the virus.

The other mothers would tell me about their children with croup coughing to the point of gagging and vomiting, coughing all night unable to sleep, and coughing themselves into fits of tears that only worsened the coughing. Though he remained ill for a couple days, my son did not cough again after being treated in the emergency room, and the stridor did not return. He recovered from his croup quite quickly, but I did not. When he was not next to me in bed the baby monitor was pressed to my ear again and I did not sleep well for months.

What kind of word, my husband wanted to know, was croup? He thought it sounded archaic, like something children used to suffer from long ago. The origin of the word, I discovered, is the sound of the cough itself, and in its definition I found the ghost that continued to haunt me: "An inflammatory disease of the larynx and trachea of children, marked by a peculiar sharp ringing cough, and frequently proving fatal in a short time." It was exactly this possibility, *fatal in a short time*, that had been keeping me up at night. But the online edition of the *Oxford English Dictionary*, with its examples from 1765 and 1866, was referring to the variety of croup that had defined the condition from Homer's ancient Greece into the twentieth century. That croup, the kind that was frequently fatal in a short time, was caused by diphtheria and has virtually disappeared in this country since the introduction of the diphtheria vaccine in the 1930s. My son had viral croup, once distinguished from diphtheria by the French with the term *faux-croup*. While diphtheria kills as many as 20 percent of the children who contract it, faux-croup is rarely fatal.

"Antibiotics, vaccines, they're both like time travel," a friend wrote to me that spring. "You go back in time and you're able to prevent a catastrophe, but who knows how you have irrevocably altered the future? I love my babies, and I go back in time (vaccinate) in order to prevent the catastrophe I can see, but then I risk the catastrophe I can't see." This was my friend who writes science fiction poetry, of course. And I knew what she meant. I had seen an episode of *Star Trek* in which the starship *Enterprise* travels through a rift in space-time and encounters an older ship that was destroyed many years earlier. Suddenly, rather than being a peacetime ship on an exploratory mission, the *Enterprise* of the present becomes a warship on the verge of a final loss to the Klingons. Because this new reality replaces the former reality instantaneously, only one crew member with a unique relationship to time understands that something has gone wrong. There are supposed to be children on the ship, she explains to the captain, and there is not supposed to be a war. When the ship from the past learns that they may prevent the current war from ever beginning by returning to the past, they heroically return to the past to die.

Every day with a child, I have discovered, is a kind of time travel. I cast my mind ahead with each decision I make, wondering what I might be giving or taking from my child in the future. I send him off to preschool, where he learns about germs and rules, wondering all the time who he might have been if he had not learned to wash his hands and stand in line as soon as he could talk. But even when I do nothing, I am aware that I am irrevocably changing the future. Time marches forward in a course that is forever altered by the fact that I did nothing.

For several nights while my son had croup I sat with him for most of the night, holding him upright while he slept so that he could breathe more easily. There was nothing else I could do for him. I traveled back in time then, or so I felt, passing through a space-time rift into what I imagined might have been the experience of a mother a hundred years ago, when faux-croup could just as easily have been killing croup. I thought of the mothers in Daniel Defoe's *A Journal of the Plague Year*, who were said to have died after losing their children—not of the plague, but of grief.

¶ "The Circassian women," Voltaire wrote to the French in 1733, "have, from time immemorial, communicated the smallpox to their children when not above six months old by making an incision in the arm, and by putting into this incision a pustule, taken carefully from the body of another child." It was women who inoculated their children, and Voltaire mourned the fact that the "lady of some French ambassador" had not brought it from Constantinople to Paris. "What prompted the Circassians to introduce this custom, which seems so strange to others," Voltaire wrote, "is a motive common to all: maternal love and self-interest."

Medical care was still mainly the domain of women then, though the tradition of the female healer was already threatened by physicians and the Church. Midwives and wise women, guilty of crimes that included providing contraception and easing the pains of labor, were particularly persecuted in the witch hunts that burned across Europe from the fifteenth to the eighteenth century. According to the Catholic Church's official guide for witch hunters, midwives belonged to the class of good witches who healed and did not harm, but this made them no less witches.

While women were being executed for their suspicious ability to heal the sick, physicians in European universities studied Plato and Aristotle but learned very little about the body. They did not experiment, did not practice science as we know it, and had little empirical data to support their treatments, which were often superstitious in nature. Wise women were themselves susceptible to superstition, but as far back as the early middle ages they used ergot to speed contractions and belladonna to prevent miscarriage. Saint Hildegarde of Bingen cataloged the healing properties of 213 medicinal plants, and women lay healers knew of recipes for effective painkillers and anti-inflammatories at a time when physicians were still writing prayers on the jaws of their patients to heal toothaches.

Benjamin Rush, one of the fathers of American medicine, bled his patients to, as Barbara Ehrenreich and Deirdre English put it, "Transylvanian excesses." In the late eighteenth and early nineteenth century, patients were bled to a faint, dosed with mercury, and blistered with mustard plasters. While medical schools excluded women from formal medical education, physicians competed, sometimes aggressively, with their informal practice in the home. But the art of healing, as doctors would discover, is rather difficult to commodify. The wise practice of waiting and watching is hard to sell, in part because it looks a lot like doing nothing. The pressures of the marketplace, Ehrenreich and English suggest, led to the practice of "heroic" medicine, which relied heavily on dangerous therapies like bleeding. The purpose of heroic medicine was not so much to heal the patient as it was to produce some measurable, and ideally dramatic, effect for which the patient could be billed. Dr. Rush, for one, was accused of killing more patients than he cured.

Childbirth was one of the last areas of health care to be claimed by physicians. Modesty and tradition stood in the way of men attending births, so obstetricians sold their services through publicity campaigns that cast midwives as ignorant, dirty, and dangerous. In the nineteenth century, poor urban women could give birth in charity hospitals for free, though wealthier women still gave birth at home. As childbirth moved into hospitals, the maternal death rate rose dramatically. Childbed fever, as puerperal sepsis was called, was spread by doctors who did not wash their hands between exams. But doctors blamed it on tight petticoats, fretting, and bad morals.

In the twentieth century, psychologists blamed schizophrenia on overbearing mothers who smothered their children. Homosexuality, categorized as a mental illness until 1973, was blamed on anxious mothers who coddled their children. Autism, according to the prevailing theory of the 1950s, was blamed on cold, insensitive "refrigerator mothers." Even now, mothers provide "a convenient missing link in germ theory," as the psychotherapist Janna Malamud Smith observes. "If it is not viral or bacterial," she quips, "it must be maternal."

In 1998, the British gastroenterologist Andrew Wakefield proposed a theory that suggested pharmaceutical companies, rather than mothers, were causing autism. The publication in the *Lancet* of his now retracted case study of twelve children was accompanied by a promotional video and a press conference, in which Wakefield supported the suspicions of parents who already believed vaccines were unsafe. His paper speculated that the MMR vaccine might be linked to a behavioral syndrome that included symptoms of autism. While the publicity around Wakefield's paper precipitated a dramatic drop in vaccination against measles, the paper itself concluded, "We did not prove an association between measles, mumps, and rubella vaccine and the syndrome described," and the primary finding was that more research was needed.

Over the next decade, study after study would fail to find a link between the MMR vaccine and autism, and even researchers sympathetic to Wakefield's hypothesis were unable to replicate his work. In 2004, an investigative journalist discovered that Wakefield had been paid for his research by a lawyer preparing a lawsuit against a vaccine manufacturer. And in 2007, Britain's

General Medical Council launched an investigation into Wakefield's ethics that concluded with the decision that his conduct was "irresponsible and dishonest," that he had subjected children to unnecessary invasive procedures, and that he had "repeatedly breached fundamental principles of research medicine." Wakefield could no longer practice medicine in Britain, but he had already emigrated to the United States. "This is the way the system deals with dissent," Wakefield would say of the verdict, which he refashioned as persecution. His research was being suppressed, he insisted, because he had dared to listen to parents, "in particular the association parents made with the vaccine."

Even a modestly informed woman squinting at the rough outlines of a compressed history of medicine can discern that quite a bit of what has passed for science in the past two hundred years, particularly where women are concerned, has not been the product of scientific inquiry so much as it has been the refuse of science repurposed to support already existing ideologies. In this tradition, Wakefield's study forwarded a hypothesis that was already in the air, a hypothesis that held particular appeal for women still haunted by the legacy of the refrigerator mother theory. Those who went on to use Wakefield's inconclusive work to support the notion that vaccines cause autism are not guilty of ignorance or science denial so much as they are guilty of using weak science as it has always been used—to lend false credibility to an idea that we want to believe for other reasons.

Believing that vaccination causes devastating diseases allows us to tell ourselves a story we already know: what heals may harm and the sum of science is not always progress. "Women know very well that knowledge from the natural sciences has been used in the interests of our domination and not our liberation," Donna Haraway writes. And this understanding, she observes, can render us less vulnerable to the seductive claims of absolute truth that are sometimes made in the name of science. But it can also invite us to undervalue the place and importance of scientific knowledge. We need science, Haraway warns. Where it is not built on social domination, science can be liberating.

¶ It is difficult to read any historical account of small-pox without encountering the word *filth*. In the nineteenth century, smallpox was widely considered a disease of filth, which meant that it was largely understood to be a disease of the poor. According to filth theory, any number of contagious diseases were caused by bad air that had been made foul by excrement or rot. The sanitary conditions of the urban poor threatened the middle class, who shuttered their windows against the air blowing off the slums. Filth, it was thought, was responsible not just for disease, but also for immorality. "Unclean! Unclean!" the heroine of *Dracula* laments when she discovers she has been bitten by the vampire, and her despair is for the fate of her soul as much as the fate of her body.

Filth theory was eventually replaced by germ theory, a superior understanding of the nature of contagion, but filth theory was not entirely wrong or useless. Raw sewage running in the streets can certainly spread diseases, though smallpox is not one of them, and the sanitation reforms inspired by filth theory dramatically reduced the incidence of cholera, typhus, and plague. Clean drinking water was among the most significant of those reforms. The reversal of the Chicago River, for instance, so that the sewage dumped into that river was not delivered directly to Lake Michigan, the city's drinking water supply, had some obvious benefits for the citizens of Chicago.

Long after the reversal of that river, the mothers I meet on the beaches of Lake Michigan do not worry much over filth. Most of us believe that dirt is good for our kids, but some of us are wary of the grass in the parks, which may or may not have been treated with toxic chemicals. The idea that toxins, rather than filth or germs, are the root cause of most maladies is a popular theory of disease among people like me. The toxins that concern us range from pesticide residue to high fructose corn syrup, and particularly suspect substances include the bisphenol A lining our tin cans, the phthalates in our shampoos, and the chlorinated Tris in our couches and mattresses.

I already practiced some intuitive toxicology before my pregnancy, but I became thoroughly immersed in it after my son was born. As long as a child takes only breast milk, I discovered, one can enjoy the illusion of a closed system, a body that is not yet in dialogue with the impurities of farm and factory. Caught up in the romance of the untainted body, I remember feeling agony when my son drank water for the first time. "Unclean! Unclean!" my mind screamed.

"He was too pure," a Baltimore mother said of her son, who developed leukemia as an infant. His mother blamed the pollutants in vaccines for his illness, and herself for allowing him to be vaccinated. Fears that formaldehyde from vaccines may cause cancer are similar to fears of mercury and aluminum, in that they coalesce around minuscule amounts of the substance in question, amounts considerably smaller than amounts from other common sources of exposure to the same substance. Formaldehyde is in automobile exhaust and cigarette smoke, as well as paper bags and paper towels, and it is released by gas stoves and open fireplaces. Many vaccines contain traces of the formaldehyde used to inactivate viruses, and this can be alarming to those of us who associate formaldehyde with dead frogs in glass jars. Large concentrations are indeed toxic, but formaldehyde is a product of our bodies, essential to our metabolism, and the amount of formaldehyde already circulating in our systems is considerably greater than the amount we receive through vaccination.

As for mercury, a child will almost certainly get more mercury exposure from her immediate environment than from vaccination. This is true, too, of the aluminum that is often used as an adjuvant in vaccines to intensify the immune response. Aluminum is in a lot of things, including fruits and cereals as well as, again, breast milk. Our breast milk, it turns out, is as polluted as our environment at large. Laboratory analysis of breast milk has detected paint thinners, dry-cleaning fluids, flame retardants, pesticides, and rocket fuel. "Most of these chemicals are found in microscopic amounts," the journalist Florence Williams notes, "but if human milk were sold at the local Piggly Wiggly, some stock would exceed federal foodsafety levels for DDT residues and PCBs."

The definition of *toxin* can be somewhat surprising if you have grown accustomed to hearing the word in the context of flame retardants and parabens. Though *toxin* is now often used to refer to man-made chemicals, the most precise meaning of the term is still reserved for biologically produced poisons. The pertussis toxin, for example, is responsible for damage to the lungs that can cause whooping cough to linger for months after the bacteria that produce it have been killed by antibiotics. The diphtheria toxin is a poison potent enough to cause massive organ failure, and tetanus produces a deadly neurotoxin. Vaccination now protects us against all these toxins.

Toxoid is the term for a toxin that has been rendered no longer toxic, but the existence of a class of vaccines called toxoids probably does not help quell widespread concerns that vaccination is a source of toxicity. The consumer advocate Barbara Loe Fisher routinely supports these fears, referring to vaccines as "biologicals of unknown toxicity" and calling for nontoxic preservatives and more studies on the "toxicity of all other vaccine additives" and their potential "cumulative toxic effects." The toxicity she speaks of is elusive, shifting from the biological components of the vaccines to their preservatives, then to an issue of accumulation that implicates not just vaccines, but also toxicity from the environment at large.

In this context, fear of toxicity strikes me as an old anxiety with a new name. Where the word *filth* once suggested, with its moralist air, the evils of the flesh, the word *toxic* now condemns the chemical evils of our industrial world. This is not to say that concerns over environmental pollution are not justified—like filth theory, toxicity theory is anchored in legitimate dangers —but that the way we think about toxicity bears some resemblance to the way we once thought about filth. Both theories allow their subscribers to maintain a sense of control over their own health by pursuing personal purity. For the filth theorist, this meant a retreat into the home, where heavy curtains and shutters might seal out the smell of the poor and their problems. Our version of this shuttering is now achieved through the purchase of purified water, air purifiers, and food produced with the promise of purity.

Purity, especially bodily purity, is the seemingly innocent concept behind a number of the most sinister social actions of the past century. A passion for bodily purity drove the eugenics movement that led to the sterilization of women who were blind, black, or poor. Concerns for bodily purity were behind miscegenation laws that persisted more than a century after the abolition of slavery, and behind sodomy laws that were only recently declared unconstitutional. Quite a bit of human solidarity has been sacrificed in pursuit of preserving some kind of imagined purity.

If we do not yet know exactly what the presence of a vast range of chemicals in umbilical cord blood and breast milk might mean for the future of our children's health, we do at least know that we are no cleaner, even at birth, than our environment at large. We are all already polluted. We have more microorganisms in our guts than we have cells in our bodies—we are crawling with bacteria and we are full of chemicals. We are, in other words, continuous with everything here on earth. Including, and especially, each other.

¶ In the first few weeks after my son was born a March wind blew off the lake and through our apartment, where I sat for hours each night in a stiff wooden rocking chair, rocking my restless baby and staring at the windows through which I could barely see the shadows of tree limbs flailing in the wind. The chair creaked and the wind moaned and I heard a tapping at the glass and a flapping around the sill and I knew a vampire was there, trying to get in. By daylight I would be reminded that a flagpole was near that window, with a flapping flag and a tapping line, but in the moment I felt terror. I was calmed only by my belief, instilled by a recent vampire movie, that the vampire could not enter without my permission.

I avoided mirrors in the dark, when I slept I woke from bloody nightmares, and I saw things moving that were not moving. During the day, I began to think the lake was singing to me. It was a single, low tone that only I could hear. I was as disquieted by this as I was comforted. I kept two tall glass liter jars of drinking water on the table next to my rocking chair. Staring at the jars as I nursed the baby I recalled being told in the hospital that I had lost two liters of blood. It remained a mystery to me how anyone could have known how much blood I lost because it went all over the floor. My husband would describe to me much later the sound it made, the lapping of small waves as the blood puddled and nurses pushed at the edges of the pool with towels. But I never saw any of it, never even heard the lapping sound, so those two glass liter jars were my only measure of what I had lost.

Vampires were in the air then. *True Blood* was a new television series and *The Vampire Diaries* was about to premiere, while the *Twilight* saga played out in a series of books I did not read followed by movies I did not see. A car parked on my block had a bumper sticker that read

Blood Is the New Black and on my first visit to the bookstore after giving birth I noticed a new section devoted exclusively to vampire novels for teenagers. Vampires were part of the cultural moment, but as a new mother I became fixated on them in part because they were a way for me to think about something else. The vampire was a metaphor, though it is hard to say whether it was a metaphor for my baby or for myself. My baby slept by day and woke at night to feed from me, sometimes drawing blood with his toothless jaws. He grew more vigorous each day, even as I remained weak and pale. But I was living off blood that was not mine.

Immediately after my son's birth, in an otherwise uncomplicated delivery, my uterus inverted, bursting capillaries and spilling blood. After giving birth without any medical intervention, without painkillers or an IV in place, I was rushed to surgery and put under general anesthesia. I woke up disoriented, shivering violently under a pile of heated blankets. "That happens to everyone who comes down here," my midwife observed from a bright and hazy place above me, inadvertently reinforcing my sense that I had, indeed, gone down to the banks of the River Styx. *Where is down here?* I kept wondering. I was too weak to move much, but when I tried I discovered that my body was lashed with tubes and wires—I had an IV in each arm, a catheter down my leg, monitors on my chest, and an oxygen mask on my face.

Alone in the recovery room, I slipped into sleep, waking with the unnerving sensation that I had stopped breathing. Machines were beeping around me. A nurse fiddled with the machines, mentioning that she thought they might be malfunctioning because they seemed to be indicating that I had stopped breathing. I coughed and could not catch my breath, struggling to say "help" before I passed out. A doctor was standing at the foot of my bed when I came to and it was decided that I would receive a transfusion. This excited the nurse, who told me that transfusions are like magic. She had seen the color come back into gray people after they had received transfusions, she said, she had seen people who could not move sit up and ask for food. Without using the words *life* or *death*, she let me know that she had seen the dead come back to life.

I did not feel like I was coming back to life as the re-frigerated blood entered my veins. I felt an ominous cold ache spreading from my arm toward my chest. "People aren't usually awake for this," the doctor said when I mentioned the temperature of the blood. He was stand-ing precariously on a stool with wheels, improvising a rig that would hold the bag of blood closer to the ceiling so that gravity would pull it into my body more quickly. By hospital policy my baby could not be in the recovery room with me and the doctor could not change that, but he could try to devise a way to get the blood into me fast-er so that I could leave the recovery room sooner. My vision began to blacken around the edges, my stomach turned, and the room spun around me. This was all nor-mal, the doctor told me. "Remember," he said, "it's not your blood."

There are many explanations for the extreme fearful-ness I felt in the weeks after my son's birth—I was a new mother, I was far from my family, I was anemic, I was delirious with fatigue. But the true source of my fear eluded me until months later, when I went out on Lake Michigan in my little canoe made of bent wood covered with a transparent canvas. I had been on the lake many times before in that boat and I had never been afraid, but this time my blood was pounding in my ears. I was newly aware of the immensity of the water under me, its vast cold depths, and I was painfully aware of the fragility of my boat. *Oh*, I thought to myself, with some disappointment, *I'm afraid of death.*

Vampires are immortal, but they are not exactly alive. *Undead* was the term Bram Stoker used for Dracula. Frankenstein and zombies and any number of animated corpses are all undead, rather than immortal in the manner of Greek gods. The term *undead* amused me in the months when I was recovering from my son's birth, a time when I frequently found reason to think of it. I was alive, and gratefully so, but I felt entirely undead.

Nitroglycerine was injected into me during the surgery that repaired my uterus. "The same thing that's used in bombs," my midwife reported. I wanted the IV lines out of my arms as soon as I left the recovery room so that I could hold my son comfortably, but the midwife explained that I needed intravenous antibiotics to prevent infection. "You've had a lot of people's hands in you," she said frankly. Some of the hands were hers, in me to help deliver the baby and the placenta, but then there was also my surgery, which was performed exclusively with human hands, leaving no incisions. When I learned this, it struck me as both magical and mundane that the technology that had saved me was simply hands. Of course, our technology is us.

You've had a lot of people's hands in you was a phrase I would hear in my mind for a long time after that surgery, along with *Remember, it's not your blood*. My pregnancy, like every pregnancy, had primed me for the understanding that my body was not mine alone and that its boundaries were more porous than I had ever been led to believe. It was not an idea that came easily, and I was dismayed by how many of the metaphors that occurred to me when I was pregnant were metaphors of political violence—invasion, occupation, and colonization. But during the birth, when the violence to my body was greatest, I was most aware not of the ugliness of a body's dependence on other bodies, but of the beauty of it. Everything that happened to me in the hospital after my son's delivery, even things I understand now as cold or brutal, I experienced at that time as aglow with humanity. Alarms were sounded for me, doctors rushed to me, bags of blood were rigged for me, ice chips were held to my lips. Human hands were in me and in everything that touched me—in the nitroglycerine, in the machines that monitored my breathing, in the blood that wasn't mine.

"If you want to understand any moment in time, or any cultural moment, just look at their vampires," says Eric Nuzum, author of *The Dead Travel Fast*. Our vampires are not like the remorseless Victorian vampires, who had a taste for the blood of babies and did not seem to feel badly about it. Our vampires are conflicted. Some of them go hungry rather than feed on humans, and some of them drink synthetic blood. "Almost all of these current vampires are struggling to be *moral*," the journalist Margot Adler observed after immersing herself in vampire novels and vampire television for months after her husband's death. "It's conventional to talk about vampires as sexual, with their hypnotic powers and their intimate penetrations and their blooddrinking and so forth," she reported. "But most of these modern vampires are not talking as much about sex as they are about power."

Power, of course, is vampiric. We enjoy it only because

someone else does not. Power is what philosophers would call a positional good, meaning that its value is determined by how much of it one has in comparison to other people. Privilege, too, is a positional good, and some have argued that health is as well.

Our vampires, whatever else they are, remain a reminder that our bodies are penetrable. A reminder that we feed off of each other, that we need each other to live. Our vampires reflect both our terrible appetites and our agonized restraint. When our vampires struggle with their need for blood, they give us a way of thinking about what we ask of each other in order to live.

¶ My father has a scar on his left arm from his small-pox vaccination more than half a century ago. That vaccine is responsible for the worldwide eradication of smallpox, with the last case of natural infection occurring in the year I was born. Three years later, in 1980, the disease that had killed more people in the twentieth century than all that century's wars was officially declared gone from Earth.

The smallpox virus now exists only in two laboratories, one in the United States and the other in Russia. Beginning shortly after the eradication of smallpox, the World Health Organization set a number of deadlines for the destruction of these stores, but neither country complied. In a 2011 discussion of the matter, the United States argued for more time with the virus so that a better vaccine could be developed, just to be safe. Smallpox has now ceased to be a disease and is only a potential weapon. And even if the last stores are destroyed, it may remain a weapon. There is plenty we do not know about small-pox, including why it is such a virulent disease, but we know enough, in theory, to resurrect it in a laboratory. "Our knowledge," Carl Zimmer observes, "gives the virus its own kind of immortality."

Thirty years after routine vaccination for smallpox ceased in the United States, the government asked researchers at the University of Iowa to test the remaining stores of the vaccine for efficacy. This was in the long moment after 9/11 when every potential terrorist attack was anticipated, including the use of smallpox as a biological weapon. The smallpox vaccine proved to be effective even after having been stored for decades and diluted to increase the supply. But the results of the vaccine trial, says Patricia Winokur, director of the university's Vaccine Research and Education Unit, were "unacceptable by today's standards." A third of the people who received the vaccine suffered serious fevers or rashes and were sick, in some cases, for several days.

That vaccine eliminated smallpox, but it remains far more dangerous than any vaccine currently on our childhood schedule. The risk of death after vaccination against smallpox, according to one estimate, is about one in a million. And the risk of hospitalization is about one in a hundred thousand. Many of the children in my father's generation took that risk. They were the generation of the Polio Pioneers, the 650,000 children from all over the country who were volunteered by their parents to test the first polio vaccine. This was after Jonas Salk had tested the vaccine on himself and his own three boys. I have seen pictures of the Polio Pioneers, schoolchildren just slightly older than my son, standing in lines with their shirtsleeves rolled up, grinning for the camera.

"They were afraid of polio and of the bomb," Jane Smith writes of their parents, "and they tended to think of them in the same terms, as sudden forces that would attack without warning and destroy their own and their children's lives." The Polio Pioneers were born in the wake of Hiroshima, to parents who had, in many cases, been enlisted into wartime service. The forms they signed to give permission for their children to receive the experimental vaccine did not ask for their consent, but allowed them to "request" to be part of the trial. It is hard to imagine parents now making that request. While we routinely call for more vaccine testing, and more human trials, the unspoken assumption is that we do not intend our children to be the subjects of those trials.

Polio is the next disease likely to be eradicated through vaccination, though that project has proved more difficult than smallpox eradication. Unlike people with smallpox, the majority of people who contract polio carry it without symptoms and never develop paralysis, but can pass the disease to others. There is no highly visible rash that can be used to identify and quarantine every case, as with smallpox, so the elimination of polio is more dependent on universal vaccination.

Polio is now endemic only in Pakistan, Afghanistan, and Nigeria. The polio eradication campaign in Nigeria came to a temporary standstill in 2003, when fears that it was a plot by Western powers to sterilize Muslim children were embraced by religious and political leaders there. "We believe that modern-day Hitlers have deliberately adulterated the oral polio vaccines with anti-fertility drugs and contaminated it with certain viruses which are known to cause HIV and AIDS," the chairman of the Supreme Council for Sharia in Nigeria maintained, urging parents to refuse vaccination.

During a time of mounting aggression against Muslim nations by the West, the anthropologist Maryam Yahya observes, Muslims in Nigeria were drawing a connection between the invasion of Iraq and Afghanistan and the invasion of their homes by door-to-door vaccinators. And because polio was endemic in a largely Muslim region of the country, the polio campaign seemed to be disproportionately targeting Muslims. There was also the uncertainty created by the fracture of the Nigerian state itself. When competing political groups tested the oral polio vaccine for the presence of an estrogen that might affect fertility, they produced different results — one found none, the other found traces. And then there was the lack of primary health care across the country. "The Nigerian people are astonished that the federal government, with the support of the international community,"

Yahya writes, "is spending huge resources on 'free' polio vaccines when basic medicines to treat even minor ailments are beyond the reach of the average person." In the push to eradicate polio, other preventable diseases like measles did not receive the same attention, even while they killed more children.

"What becomes increasingly apparent in these conversations," Yahya writes of her fieldwork in Nigeria, "is a lack of trust in the government and the West, portrayed by many as 'partners in crime.'" This mistrust, she warns, should not be dismissed, and vaccination rumors must be understood as "an idiom crystallizing valid commentary on broader political experience in colonial and post-colonial settings." By 2004, less than a year after the boycott began, Nigeria had become the center of polio transmission for the world. The disease spread into seventeen other countries including Benin, Botswana, Burkina Faso, Cameroon, the Central African Republic, Chad, Côte d'Ivoire, Ethiopia, Ghana, Guinea, Mali, Sudan, and Togo. The boycott ended after Nigerian officials approved the use of polio vaccine produced by a company based in a Muslim country.

In 2012, a Taliban leader in northern Pakistan banned polio vaccination in his region until the United States ceased drone strikes there. Vaccination campaigns, he claimed, were a form of American espionage. While resembling the rumors of secret plots in Nigeria, this was, unfortunately, more easily verifiable. In pursuit of Osama bin Laden, the CIA had used a fake vaccination campaign—administering real hep B vaccine, but not the three doses necessary for immunity—to gather DNA evidence to help verify bin Laden's location. This deception, like other acts of war, would cost the lives of women and children. The Lady Health Workers of

Pakistan, a team of over 110,000 women trained to deliver health care door-to-door, had already endured years of brutal intimidation by the Taliban and hardly needed association with the CIA. Not long after the Taliban banned immunization, nine polio vaccinators, five of them women, were murdered in a coordinated series of attacks.

Pakistan's polio campaign was suspended after the murders, but when it resumed the murders resumed in both Pakistan and Nigeria. Nine polio vaccinators were shot in Nigeria in 2013 and, as of this writing, twenty-two health care workers have been killed in Pakistan. During the suspension of the vaccination campaign, polio virus from Pakistan was discovered in sewage samples in Egypt, which had been free of polio for nearly a decade. Polio was subsequently found in Israel, Gaza, and the West Bank, and it paralyzed thirteen children in Syria. Polio's ability to spread across national borders is part of what makes vaccine refusal a viable weapon in international warfare.

In a scene from *Apocalypse Now* more frightening than anything Francis Ford Coppola conjured for his adaptation of *Dracula*, Colonel Kurtz tells the story of returning to a camp where he had helped vaccinate children against polio to find that the children's arms had been cut off. "They were there in a pile," he said, "a pile of little arms." This was the pile of little arms that was the Vietnam War, which recalled, by way of *Heart of Darkness*, the piles of human hands that were the Belgian Congo.

I would think of those little arms and those human hands when a friend of mine who was born in Vietnam during the war told me that she was exposed to Agent Orange in the womb. After coming to this country, she did not vaccinate her children as infants, for a number of reasons, including her sense that it was not safe. I disagreed with her uneasily, knowing that my understanding of safety had been forged in a life more protected than hers. I could not ask her to risk her children for the benefit of the citizens of the country that had put her in danger. The best I could do, I determined, was hope that my own child's body might help shield them from disease. If vaccination can be conscripted into acts of war, it can still be instrumental in works of love.

¶ In the spring of 1956, a five-year-old girl was hospitalized in Minamata, Japan, with difficulty walking, difficulty talking, and convulsions. Her younger sister was admitted to the hospital two days later with the same symptoms, and eight more people were soon hospitalized. In their investigation of the mysterious epidemic, health officials found that cats were having convulsions and going mad, crows were dropping out of the sky, and fish were floating in the bay. The chemical factory in Minamata was dumping wastewater contaminated with methyl mercury into the bay, where it was accumulating in the fish and shellfish people were eating. Healthy mothers were giving birth to babies with neurological damage, and thousands of people would eventually suffer mercury poisoning.

In 2013, a global treaty banning mercury was named for Minamata. The treaty ensured that mercury mines would be phased out by 2020, emissions from power plants would be controlled, and many products containing mercury—including batteries, lamps, cosmetics, and pesticides—would no longer be manufactured, imported, or exported. Everyone in the world, the director of the United Nations Environmental Program observed, stood to benefit.

One of the most noted exemptions from the ban was thimerosal, the ethyl mercury preservative used in some vaccines. The World Health Organization recommended that thimerosal be excluded from the ban in the interest of global health, and the American Academy of Pediatricians supported the recommendation. This was, as two members of the AAP would observe, a "significant reversal" of their position in 1999, when they called for the removal of thimerosal from childhood vaccines in this country. This reversal would trigger accusations that the United States was comfortable with mercury in other people's vaccines, but not its own. The implication was that the United States was subjecting the rest of the world to its hazardous waste, which was easy to believe because it was true in other contexts.

The AAP's 1999 statement recommended suspending the use of thimerosal while its safety was evaluated, but the statement did not express much concern about the preservative. Thimerosal, as the AAP noted, had been used in vaccines since the 1930s. There was little evidence to suggest that thimerosal was dangerous, but there was also little evidence, at the time, to suggest that it was safe. A broader review of mercury exposure was under way, and the AAP made its statement shortly after the FDA found that a child's total ethyl mercury exposure from the full vaccination schedule could potentially exceed a federal limit for methyl mercury, the kind of mercury that had caused poisonings in Minamata. Subsequent research revealed "profound differences" between ethyl and methyl mercury, one of the most significant being that ethyl mercury is not associated with the neurotoxic effects of methyl mercury. Reflecting on the research that had been conducted in the thirteen years since the AAP's statement on thimerosal, a 2012 article in *Pediatrics* concluded, "There is no credible scientific evidence that the use of thimerosal in vaccines presents any risk to human health."

In 120 countries, vaccines containing thimerosal are currently used to save an estimated 1.4 million lives every year. Thimerosal is essential for multidose vaccines, which are less expensive to produce, store, and ship than single-dose vaccines. Some countries rely on multidose vaccines, not just because they are more cost effective and produce less waste than singledose vaccines, but also because they do not require refrigeration. There are places, mostly in poorer countries, where a ban on thimerosal would effectively be a ban on vaccination against diphtheria, pertussis, hep B, and tetanus.

If we knew then what we know now, the former president of the AAP has suggested, the 1999 policy on thimerosal would never have been written. Maybe so, though the AAP statement was made in response not just to a lack of data on thimerosal, but also to the social climate at the time. Andrew Wakefield's 1998 study linking the MMR vaccine to autism was causing a cascade of panic, adding to the alarm that had already been raised by a 1981 study that suggested the diphtheria-tetanus-pertussis vaccine caused brain damage. Subsequent studies in England, Denmark, and the United States had refuted that conclusion, but no new findings could un-ring the bell. The AAP statement, an effort to preserve confidence in vaccines, would eventually be used to export American anxieties.

In the event of a pandemic, thimerosal, which allows for more rapid production and distribution of vaccines, might yet be as essential in this country as it is in other countries. For now, we use expensive single-dose vaccines for the same reason many other wealthy countries do—because we can. SafeMinds, an autism advocacy group that was among the most vocally opposed to the exemption for thimerosal in the Minamata treaty, repeatedly suggested that the exemption was motivated by money. It was, in the sense that it was informed by the need for affordable vaccination in low-income countries. The groups that opposed the exemption, as global health researchers would observe in *Pediatrics*, were all nongovernmental groups like SafeMinds from high-income countries where vaccination rates would not be affected by a ban on thimerosal. Wealthier countries have the luxury of entertaining fears the rest of the world cannot afford.

¶ "Capital," Karl Marx wrote, "is dead labor, that, vampire-like, only lives by sucking living labor, and lives the more, the more labor it sucks." Vampires sucked the blood of the sleeping in ancient Greece and spread plague in medieval Europe, but after the industrial revolution, novels began to feature a new kind of vampire, the well-dressed gentleman who would become an enduring emblem of capitalism. During his 2012 presidential campaign, venture capitalist Mitt Romney, whose status as living or undead was the subject of some sporting debate, frequently found himself compared to a vampire. After transforming into a "vulture capitalist" in the primaries, he became a full-fledged vampire capitalist in Barack Obama's campaign ads. "It was like a vampire," a steelworker said of the company Romney cofounded, Bain Capital. "It came in and sucked the life out of us."

The idea of an ambitious vampire sucking the life out of honest workers resonated in a country where the value had so recently been sucked out of nearly every home. Vampirism was behind a housing crisis set off by a rash of predatory loans to home owners who lacked the ability to repay them. These loans, bundled and sold to investors, came to be known as "toxic assets" when they lost their value.

The understanding that capital can itself be toxic leads, almost inevitably, to a fear of capitalism polluting every endeavor. At the close of the 2009 H1N1 influenza pandemic, when it was clear that the flu had not caused the high mortality rates health officials had initially feared, the chair of the health committee for the Council of Europe accused the World Health Organization of colluding with pharmaceutical companies and creating a "false pandemic" to sell vaccines. The WHO met this accusation with equanimity, their spokeswoman saying,

"Criticism is part of an outbreak cycle." The WHO then invited twenty-five independent influenza experts from twenty-four countries to evaluate its actions during the pandemic.

In reading the report prepared by these experts, I paused for a long moment over a passage proposing that a fund be established to provide for the child care needs of WHO workers who could expect to be called away in the event of a pandemic. This passage was just an aside, a minor logistical note, but what caused me to pause was the evocation, for a moment, of the lived lives behind the effort to control disease. It is easy to forget that an organization known as the "WHO" is composed of actual individuals, with children and child care concerns like my own.

The independent experts found no evidence that commercial interests had influenced the WHO or attempted to influence it, and no evidence that the WHO had wrongfully exaggerated the pandemic. Their report explained that one of the reasons certain precautions taken by the WHO could seem, in hindsight, out of proportion with the actual threat posed by the pandemic is that the organization had been preparing for a possible outbreak of avian influenza H5N1, a highly lethal strain, and initial reports had suggested that the fatality rate of H1N1 might also be quite high. "Influenza viruses are notoriously unpredictable," the chairman of the committee noted in his introduction to the report, adding that we were "lucky" this time. "In the Committee's view," the report concluded, "the inference by some critics that invisible commercial influences must account for WHO's actions ignores the power of the core public-health ethos to prevent disease and save lives."

The extent to which it is hard to imagine an ethos

powerful enough to compete with capitalism, even if that ethos is based on the inherent value of human lives, is suggestive of how successfully capitalism has limited our imaginations. "Occupy immune systems," a friend joked when she heard I was writing about vaccination, but I did not immediately recognize the joke and spent some time searching the web for an organization called Occupy Immune Systems. The possibility did not seem unlikely. At that moment, the Occupy movement was carrying the declaration "We are the 99%" from Wall Street to Chicago to San Francisco, rapidly becoming an ongoing global protest of capitalism.

Immunity is a public space. And it can be occupied by those who choose not to carry immunity. For some of the mothers I know, a refusal to vaccinate falls under a broader resistance to capitalism. But refusing immunity as a form of civil disobedience bears an unsettling resemblance to the very structure the Occupy movement seeks to disrupt—a privileged 1 percent are sheltered from risk while they draw resources from the other 99 percent.

Dracula, published shortly after the third and final volume of Marx's *Capital*, is fairly easily subjected to Marxist interpretation. "Like capital, Dracula is impelled towards a continuous growth," the literary critic Franco Moretti writes, "an unlimited expansion of his domain: accumulation is inherent in his nature." What makes Dracula terrifying, Moretti argues, is not that he likes blood or enjoys blood, but that he needs blood.

The drive toward capital, as *Dracula* suggests, is inherently inhumane. We are justified in feeling threatened by the unlimited expansion of industry, and we are justified in fearing that our interests are secondary to corporate interests. But refusal of vaccination undermines a system that is not actually typical of capitalism. It is a system in which both the burdens and the benefits are shared across the entire population. Vaccination allows us to use the products of capitalism for purposes that are counter to the pressures of capital.

Observing that we have waged wars on poverty and drugs as well as cancer, Susan Sontag writes, "Abuse of the military metaphor may be inevitable in a capitalist society, a society that increasingly restricts the scope and credibility of appeals to ethical principle, in which it is thought foolish not to subject one's actions to the calculus of self-interest and profitability." In such a society, preventive measures to protect public health require elaborate justifications. War, Sontag suggests, is one of the few activities in which we are not expected to consider practicality and expense. Declaring a metaphorical war on a disease is how we justify the inevitable impracticalities of protecting the most vulnerable among us.

My son was three years old by the time the CDC released their estimate of how many people worldwide had died from H1N1 in 2009, when he was an infant. The death toll calculated by the CDC, somewhere between 150,000 and 575,000, made the severity of H1N1 comparable to a typical seasonal outbreak of influenza. But this flu had killed young people disproportionately. In the United States, ten times more children died of H1N1 than die in a typical flu season. Worldwide, somewhere around 9.7 million years of potential human life had been lost in the pandemic.

"Follow the money," a friend of mine says in defense of the theory that vaccination is simply a profit-driven scheme controlled by pharmaceutical companies with unchecked influence over government and medicine.

My conversation with her reminds me of Eve Sedgwick's essay on paranoia, in which she recounts a conversation with her friend Cindy Patton during the first decade of the AIDS epidemic. Sedgwick asked Patton what she thought about rumors that the HIV virus was part of a plot engineered by the US military, and Patton said she couldn't muster much interest. "I mean," Patton said, "even suppose we were sure of every element of a conspiracy: that the lives of Africans and African Americans are worthless in the eyes of the United States; that gay men and drug users are held cheap where they aren't actively hated; that the military deliberately researches ways to kill noncombatants whom it sees as enemies... Supposing we were ever so sure of all those things— what would we know then that we don't already know?"

A Nigerian barber said, of the idea that vaccines were a Western plot against Muslims, "If the White man really wanted to destroy us, there are many other easier ways to do it. They can poison our coca-cola..." I tend to agree. And I suspect that Coca-Cola, unpoisoned, is more harmful to our children than vaccination.

Just because we have enemies, Sedgwick proposes, does not mean we have to be paranoid. Our cynicism may be justified, but it is also sad. That so many of us find it entirely plausible that a vast network of researchers and health officials and doctors worldwide would willfully harm children for money is evidence of what capitalism is really taking from us. Capitalism has already impoverished the working people who generate wealth for others. And capitalism has already impoverished us culturally, robbing unmarketable art of its value. But when we begin to see the pressures of capitalism as innate laws of human motivation, when we begin to believe that everyone is owned, then we are truly impoverished.

¶ Whenever I complained of a sore throat as a child, my father would press his fingers gently behind my jawbone, checking for swollen lymph nodes. "I think you're going to be okay," he would say upon completing his examination. This was his verdict, too, when I called him from college, miserably ill with what he identified as "probably influenza." I asked him if there was anything I could do and he suggested, to my disappointment, drinking plenty of fluids. Then he recommended his grandmother's prescription for a bad cold—buttered toast dipped in warm milk. He described the way the butter floated on the surface of the milk and how comforting he found his grandmother's care. I wanted to know if there was some sort of medicine I could take, but what I needed, my father understood, was comfort. As an adult, I still never cease to feel a little surprise when a doctor reaches behind my jawbone to check for swollen nodes. I associate the tenderness of that gesture with my father's care.

Paternalism has fallen out of favor in medicine, just as the approach to fathering that depends on absolute authority no longer dominates parenting. But how we should care for other people remains a question. In his discussion of efforts to control childhood obesity, the philosopher Michael Merry defines paternalism as "interference with the liberty of another for the purposes of promoting some good or preventing some harm." This type of paternalism, he notes, is reflected in traffic laws, gun control, and environmental regulations. These are limits to liberty, even if they are benevolent. Interfering with the parenting of obese children, he argues, is not necessarily benevolent. There is risk in assigning risk. Children who are already stigmatized for their body type are further targeted. And families who are identified as "at risk" for obesity become at risk to discriminatory oversight. The prevention of risk, Merry observes, is often used to justify a coercive use of power.

Autonomy is usually imagined as the alternative to paternalism. But in what is sometimes called the "restaurant model" of medicine, the paternalism of doctors has been replaced by the consumerism of patients. We order tests and treatments from a menu based on our consumer research. And the doctor, who was a father in the paternalistic model, is now a waiter. The idea that the customer is always right, imported to medicine, is a dangerous dictum. "If you keep telling people that it's just a marketplace and that they're just clients and that the autonomy of the patient is what must be served to make them happy customers," the bioethicist Arthur Caplan warns, "then you have a collapse of professionalism in the face of consumer demand." Doctors may be tempted to give patients what we want, even when it is not good for us.

"Why does the term 'paternalism' have such bad press in medical circles?" asks physician John Lee. "Did everyone really have such a hard time with their dad that the reason seems self-evident?" He is paternalistic, Lee admits, but "in a good way." A return to paternalism, good or bad, is not the only alternative to consumerism. In a response to Merry's critique of paternalism, the educator Barbara Peterson proposes that we think of the problem of childhood obesity in terms of maternalism. Caretaking, she suggests, is not an inherent threat to liberty. From a feminist, caring framework," Peterson writes, "*liberty* is not defined as complete separation and independence from the parent." If fathering still reminds us of oppressive control, mothering might help us imagine relationships based not just on power, but also care."

If you're going to get medical care," my father says, "you're going to have to trust someone." I have called to ask his advice about a surgery my son's pediatrician has recommended. My father is happy to offer his thoughts, but he is also quick to remind me that he is not a pediatrician. He does not want to be the only doctor I am willing to trust.

He is, in fact, usually the first doctor I consult. When my son woke at dawn one morning with his face so swollen from an allergic reaction that the whites of his eyes were bulging over the irises, I called my father. Did I have to go to the emergency room, I wanted to know, or could I wait until the doctor's office opened in a couple hours? I could wait, my father assured me, and the swelling was not dangerous. *"It's just fluid,"* he said. I now repeat it's just fluid in my mind every time my son's eyes swell.

My son has unusually severe allergies, which he developed at an unusually young age. His pediatrician calls him her "outlier" because he is a statistical anomaly. By the time he turned three, his allergies had led to swelling in his nasal cavity, and this swelling had led to painful sinus infections, which we had cured with antibiotics several times, but which inevitably returned. After the third round of antibiotics, the pediatrician suggested surgery to remove his adenoids, which had swelled so much that they were completely blocking his nasal passage.

Surgery struck me as overkill, and I was not eager to have part of my son's lymphatic system removed from his body. When I researched the procedure, I was disturbed to discover that it was performed widely in the early 1900s as a kind of cure-all for childhood ailments. My father was sympathetic to my concerns. He himself no longer has his tonsils because a traveling doctor removed the tonsils of all four children in his family on a single visit. This was, at the time, a standard preventive measure against rheumatic fever, which ceased after research revealed that the dangers of the surgery outweighed its benefits. As a rule, it is wise to be wary of overtreatment, my father told me. But if the alternative to surgery in my son's case was the ongoing use of antibiotics or other drugs, surgery might be the more conservative option.

I delayed making a decision for well over six months, all the while trying everything else. A friend suggested an expensive air filter, which I bought. The allergist recommended that I keep our floors clean, a Sisyphean task, considering that microscopic allergens were constantly circulating through the air and settling on the floors. But I mopped the invisible dirt and I changed my son's sheets and pillowcases daily. Despite his protests, I flushed his sinuses with salt water every evening. I gave him a prescription nasal spray. I fed him raw honey and nettle tea. Then his breathing, already loud, became irregular at night. I crouched next to his bed, holding my own breath during the pauses in his breathing to gauge how long he was going without air. After particularly long pauses he woke, gasping and coughing. I scheduled the surgery.

The surgeon reminded me, on the day of the surgery, not to expect dramatic or instantaneous results. She had already been over this with me, and had already warned me that my son might continue to get infections despite the surgery. I was most hopeful not that the surgery would enact a miracle, but that it would simply do no harm. It was an easy, routine surgery, she assured me. The most dangerous part was the anesthesia.

While we waited in a room full of toy stethoscopes and toy syringes, the anesthesiologist arrived and asked if I had any questions. I told him that I would like to be with my son while he was put under and while he came back to consciousness. The doctor stiffened at this suggestion. Studies had shown, he told me, that the body language and facial expressions of anxious mothers can cause children to fear surgery and resist anesthesia. It seemed there were two ways to interpret those findings, I told him—one could determine that the mother's presence is not good for the child, or one could conclude that ensuring the confidence of the mother is essential to the well-being of the child. We began to argue in low voices, while my husband and my son applied toy bandages to each other on the other side of the room. The implication that I was a hysterical woman and a threat to my child was making me so angry that it seemed possible I might actually become hysterical. Finally, we compromised. I would be allowed to hold my son's hand while he was put under anesthesia if I agreed to position myself so that he could not see my face.

In the operating room I talked to my son from beyond his range of vision until the anesthesia took effect. Watching the muscle tone leave his face and body was disturbing, like seeing a rehearsal of death, and I was eager to go back to the waiting room as soon as he was unconscious but the anesthesiologist called after me. "Don't you want to give him a kiss?" he asked, to my disgust.

A smiley-face balloon bobbed mutely against the ceiling of the waiting room. It had been trailing us ever since my husband untied it from the stuffed pig that was given to my son by the child life specialist, who assured me that the pig could accompany my son into surgery. All the doctors were very pleased about this, even the stern surgeon. They seemed convinced that the pig would be a source of great comfort to my son.

Perhaps as a punishment intended for me, or perhaps as the result of an error or just a matter of routine, my son woke from anesthesia before I was summoned to the recovery room. I could hear him screaming "Mama! Where's my mama?" all the way down the hallway. I knew from my own experience with surgery that the moment before anesthesia takes effect and the moment after it loses effect can seem to be the same moment— in my son's mind I had vanished. When I reached him, he was thrashing in confused panic, trying to rip the IV line out of his body. I climbed up on the gurney to hold him and stroke his hair and keep his hands away from his IV while he wailed. "He won't remember any of this," the anesthesiologist assured me nervously. I was busy calming my son, but I looked up just long enough to say, "I will."

My father suggests that the time has come for another version of *Dracula* in which the vampire serves as a metaphor for medicine. Because, he says, "medicine sucks the blood out of people in a lot of ways." The cost of my son's surgery, which was considerably more than the cost of his birth, would have made it an impossible decision for many families. I was reminded of this in the days immediately after the surgery, when my son's breathing became easy and quiet. He slept better, he put on weight, and he stopped getting sinus infections. I now regret waiting to give him the surgery, but my husband does not. It was responsible of us, he says, to be skeptical.

Either despite or because of his training, my father is himself fairly skeptical of medicine. He once joked about the two-sentence textbook he would like to write for physicians: "Most problems will get better if left alone. Those problems that do not get better if left alone are likely to kill the patient no matter what you do." This is as much an argument for preventive medicine as it is a sigh of defeat.

I remain grateful for my son's surgery, just as I remain furious with the anesthesiologist and dismayed with myself for trusting my child to someone I did not myself trust. "Where there is trust, paternalism is unnecessary," the philosopher Mark Sagoff writes. "Where there is no trust, it is unconscionable." And so we are caught in a double bind.

¶ The magazines I paged through in my midwife's waiting room when I was pregnant with my son ran advertisements for disturbing little sculptures that could be made from ultrasound images of my developing fetus, as well as ads for the equally mystifying services of private cord blood banks. My midwife had already informed me that I could donate my son's cord blood to a public bank where it would be available for transplants in people with leukemia and lymphoma, among other conditions. The private banks advertised in magazines were offering, at a cost, to preserve my child's blood not for anyone who needed it, but exclusively for my child or a close relative. It was banking against future knowledge, I would discover, since the ways in which having access to one's own cord blood might be advantageous later in life are still fairly limited in practice and promising only in theory.

Interested in the transformation of a public fund into a private account, the hoarding for unknown future benefit of something that could be donated for known benefit now, I tore an ad for a private cord blood bank out of a pregnancy magazine shortly after my son's birth. That ad features a large photo of a sleeping infant next to an advice column titled "Ask Dr. Sears", with the question "Should I bank my baby's cord blood?" The response from the expert, Robert Sears, is unsurprising, considering that the advice column is actually an advertisement and Sears is a consultant for the cord blood bank being advertised. "As new treatments develop," Sears writes, "having cord blood on hand may be invaluable." The fine print at the bottom of the ad clarifies his equivocation: "There is no guarantee that treatments being studied in the laboratory or in clinical trials will be available in the future."

I had not yet read Sears's best seller, *The Vaccine Book*, when I tore out this ad. But I recognized the Sears brand, I had seen Sears endorsements on products for infants, and I knew that Robert Sears, or "Dr. Bob," as he calls himself, was the son of William Sears, a popular source of parenting advice and probably the most well known pediatrician in the United States. The widespread appeal of *The Vaccine Book*, I would come to understand, lies mainly in the compromise it offers between vaccinating and not vaccinating. For parents who fear both vaccines and infectious diseases, Sears offers two clear courses of action. One is "Dr. Bob's Selective Vaccine Schedule," a plan that provides only the vaccines Dr. Bob deems most important— leaving children unvaccinated against hep B, polio, measles, mumps, and rubella. The other is "Dr. Bob's Complete Alternative Vaccine Schedule," a plan that provides all the vaccines a child typically receives in two years on the standard schedule, but spread out over the course of eight years.

"It's the best of both worlds of disease prevention and safe vaccination," Dr. Bob writes of the alternative schedule. Because the schedule delays some vaccinations that are intended specifically to protect very young children, it is unlikely to offer the best of disease prevention. And it is unlikely to offer the best of safe vaccination in that there is no credible evidence, beyond Dr. Bob's personal speculations, that spacing and delaying vaccinations minimizes the incidence of side effects. The alternative schedule is, optimistically, the *most* of both worlds. By following this schedule, parents can secure most of the benefits of disease protection—though not at the most crucial age for that protection—while risking all of the potential side effects of vaccination.

The extra time and trouble required to follow Dr.

Bob's alternative schedule are hard to justify unless the dangers of contracting infectious diseases early in life are minimized and the dangers of vaccinating early in life are exaggerated. Much of *The Vaccine Book* is devoted to this minimization and exaggeration. Tetanus is not a disease that affects infants, according to Dr. Bob, Hib disease is rare, and measles is not that bad. He does not mention that tetanus kills hundreds of thousands of babies in the developing world every year, that most children will encounter the bacteria that causes Hib disease within the first two years of their lives, and that measles has killed more children than any other disease in history.

The idea of a middle ground on vaccination is appealing, if elusive. Competing claims to expertise countered by accusations of conflicts of interest have bred a hunger for the kind of impartial authority Dr. Bob promises in the preface to his book. But *The Vaccine Book* is not even-handed so much as it is equivocal. "Vaccines don't cause autism," Dr. Bob writes, "except when they do." And he concludes his discussion of the lack of evidence supporting a causal relationship between vaccines and certain side effects by asserting, "I'm sure the truth of the matter is somewhere between causality and coincidence."

What it might mean for a vaccine to neither cause an effect nor be simply coincidentally associated with it is unclear. There are a number of indirect side effects associated with vaccines. The measles-mumps-rubella vaccine, for example, can cause a high fever that may then cause a seizure in an infant who is prone to febrile seizures. It is the fever, not the vaccine, that causes the seizure—and the same child would be likely to suffer a seizure from a fever brought on by natural infection—but most discussions of vaccine side effects, including Dr. Bob's, do not bother with this distinction. Indirect causation is typically considered causation. And so it is here, between causality and coincidence, that I begin to fear Dr. Bob's middle ground may be a fictive location.

Dr. Bob maintains his middle ground in part by recalibrating the conversation around vaccination so that positions more cautious than his appear extreme. "I'm not sure where this hard line comes from," he writes of pediatricians who dismiss from their practices families who refuse to vaccinate their children. As Dr. Bob is probably aware, some pediatricians do not treat unvaccinated children because of the possibility that those children might expose infants in their waiting rooms to diseases that those infants are too young to be vaccinated against. In fact, the unvaccinated child who returned from a trip to Switzerland in 2008 with a case of measles that infected eleven other children was Dr. Bob's patient. It was under Dr. Bob's care that he was not vaccinated, though it was not in Dr. Bob's waiting room that he spread measles to three babies too young to be vaccinated.

"I was NOT the pediatrician who saw the measles patient and let him sit in my office," he wrote of the incident. "I was not involved in that at all." When pressed, he added, "I have simply been the family's pediatrician over the years, but I practice far away from them, so they went to a local ped for THIS problem." In Dr. Bob's world, another doctor's waiting room is not his concern and public health is entirely independent of individual health. "This is an important vaccine from a public health standpoint," he writes of the hep B vaccine, "but it's not as critical from an individual point of view." In order for this to make sense, one must believe that individuals are not part of the public.

Public health, Dr. Bob suggests, is not *our* health. "It is safe to say that we don't give this vaccine in order to protect each individual child from catching polio," Dr. Bob writes of the polio vaccine. "Rather, we do it to protect our nation as a whole in the event an outbreak does occur." As he acknowledges, "If we stop using this vaccine, polio may come back. Anyone who is over fifty knows just how scary that would be." He himself is too young to remember polio. And he has never treated a child with diphtheria or tetanus. "Hopefully, someday we will have a better way to know for sure which side effects are truly vaccine related," he writes. He is banking against future knowledge, again—using the limitless promise of scientific discovery to disguise a gamble as a prudent investment.

¶ My grandfather lost his father to tuberculosis when he was ten. On the other side of my family, both my grandmother and my grandfather lost siblings to infectious diseases. One family lost a toddler to measles and a teenager to sepsis, and the other family lost a toddler to pertussis and a teenager to tetanus. When my father was a boy, his brother was bedridden for six months with rheumatic fever. He lived, but he suffered permanent heart damage and died young of heart failure.

My father was vaccinated against five diseases as a child. I was vaccinated against seven, and my son has been vaccinated against fourteen. The proliferation of childhood vaccines has become, for some of us, a kind of metaphor for American excess. *Too many*, *too soon*, one of the slogans common to vaccine activism, could easily be a critique of just about any aspect of our modern lives.

The smallpox vaccine my father received contained far more immunizing proteins, or active ingredient, so to speak, than any of the vaccines we use today. These proteins are what the immune system is reacting to when it responds to a vaccine. In that sense, a single dose of the smallpox vaccine our parents received presented a greater challenge to the immune system than the total challenge presented by all the twenty-six immunizations for fourteen diseases we now give to our children over the course of two years.

When asked by his colleagues to address the question of whether too many vaccines are given too early in life, the pediatrician Paul Offit set out to quantify the capacity of the infant immune system, which is already known to be quite impressive. Infants are exposed to an onslaught of bacteria the moment they leave the womb, even before they exit the birth canal. Any infant who does not live in a bubble is likely to find the everyday work of fighting off infection more taxing than process-ing weakened antigens from multiple immunizations.

Offit is a professor of pediatrics at the University of Pennsylvania and the head of the Division of Infectious Diseases at the Children's Hospital of Philadelphia. He is the coinventor of a vaccine, the author of several books about vaccination, and a former member of the CDC's advisory committee on immunization practices. He is also, if you believe the Internet, a "Devil's servant" known as "Dr. Proffit." He earned this distinction, along with some credible death threats, by being an outspoken advocate for vaccination.

Offit is associated with the devil on a website that also compiles evidence that the Holocaust was a hoax and that anti-Semitism was invented by Zionists as a justification for the creation of Israel. Accusations that Offit is a "vaccine profiteer" are generated by a blogger named J. B. Handley, himself no stranger to profit. Handley, a venture capitalist, is the cofounder of a private equity firm with over $1 billion under manage-ment as well as the cofounder of Generation Rescue, an autism advocacy organization.

In his book *Autism's False Prophets*, Offit explores the problematic history of the theory that vaccines cause autism while detailing the research refuting that theory. The question of whether vaccines cause autism is not, Offit makes clear, the subject of any ongoing scientific debate. And groups like Generation Rescue, he reveals, spend a lot of money spreading misinformation and pro-moting ineffective therapies. Some parents of autistic children consider this exploitation. Meanwhile, Offit receives email messages reading, "I will hang you by your neck until you are dead!"

"It's hurtful," Offit says of the persistent suggestion

that his research has been driven by profit. He also finds it somewhat laughable. "Who ever goes into science," he asks, "thinking, *God, if I could just figure out which of these two viral surface proteins evoke neutralizing antibodies, I'll be rich beyond my wildest dreams!*" He would have made a much better salary, he observes, if he had gone into private practice as a pediatrician after medical school rather than going into research.

When Offit was an intern, he saw a nine-month-old baby die of rotavirus. He had not realized, until that moment, that children died of rotavirus in the United States. After his internship, he joined a team of researchers who were working toward a potential vaccine to protect against rotavirus, which caused the hospitalization of 70,000 children in the United States and killed over 600,000 children in the developing world every year. This was in 1981, and the chance that their work would result in a vaccine was only a remote possibility at that point.

"It took us ten years," Offit says, "to answer the question, *How can we give a vaccine that induces an immune response but doesn't cause disease?* Then we went to a series of companies, because only pharmaceutical companies have the resources and expertise to make a vaccine. In addition, no pharmaceutical company will advance a technology that is not protected. We had to patent it." Even after the vaccine was patented, there was no certainty it would ever be marketed.

Over the course of sixteen years, the RotaTeq vaccine was tested for safety in progressively larger groups of children. The final safety trial involved over 70,000 children in twelve countries and cost Merck about $350 million. When the vaccine was licensed, Children's Hospital sold the patent for $182 million. The hospital

118

owns the intellectual property of its researchers, so 90 percent of this money went to the hospital and was put back into research. The remaining 10 percent was divided among the three researchers who had worked for over twenty-five years on the vaccine.

Compared to other pharmaceuticals, vaccines are costly to develop and generate modest profits. "In 2008, Merck's revenue from RotaTeq was $665 million," the journalist Amy Wallace observes. "Meanwhile, a blockbuster drug like Pfizer's Lipitor is a $12 billion-a-year business." Older vaccines make considerably less money than new vaccines, and vaccine production has not proved profitable enough to keep many companies from leaving the business over the past thirty years.

Why the success of his vaccine should render his expertise in immunology invalid remains baffling to Offit. "It's not like I invented a better way to freebase cocaine," he says. But he understands the other source of his infamy. In response to the question of how many vaccines is too many, Offit determined that a child could theoretically handle a total of 100,000 vaccines or up to 10,000 vaccines at once. He came to regret this number, though he does not believe that it is inaccurate. "The 100,000 number makes me sound like a madman," he says. "Because that's the image: 100,000 shots sticking out of you. It's an awful image."

¶ When I took my son to the doctor for his one-year checkup, I was surprised to learn that he would be vaccinated against chicken pox. He had already been vaccinated against Hib, diphtheria, hep B, and rotavirus—diseases I was entirely unfamiliar with. But chicken pox was a disease I knew and remembered well from my own childhood, when all four children in my family had it at the same time. My infant sister was not yet a year old then, I had pox in my nose and throat and ears, and my mother was home giving us baking soda baths while my father worked. I could appreciate what it might have been like for my mother to care for four sick children only after I became a mother myself, but vaccinating against chicken pox still struck me as excessive.

The pediatrician smiled generously when I asked if we could limit my son's vaccines to those that protected against diseases that could kill him. It was unlikely chicken pox would kill him, she allowed, but there were some good reasons to want to avoid the illness. Since my own childhood, there has been a rise in virulent skin infections resistant to antibiotics. Chicken pox can lead to infection with staph and Group A strep, also known as "flesh-eating" bacteria, as well as pneumonia and encephalitis. And, like most diseases, chicken pox can manifest mildly or dramatically. About 10,000 previously healthy children were hospitalized annually before the vaccine was introduced, and about 70 died every year. This was sufficient to convince me to accept the vaccine, but there was more.

Once you are infected with chicken pox, the varicella virus never leaves your body. It lives in your nerve roots and must be kept at bay by your immune system for the rest of your life. In times of stress, it can return as shingles, a painful inflammation of the nerves. The reawakened virus can cause strokes and paralysis, but the most common complication of shingles is nerve pain that persists for months or years. Immunity produced by disease, in this case, involves an ongoing relationship with the disease.

The vaccine virus that protects against chicken pox can also remain in a person's nervous system. But being a weakened virus, it is far less likely to reawaken as shingles. And when it does, it is less likely to cause a severe case of shingles. Some parents feel that the immunity produced by the chicken pox vaccine is inferior to immunity by natural infection because it does not last as long. To carry immunity through adulthood, when chicken pox can be quite serious, one must get a booster in adolescence. "So what?" my father says. I am trying to explain the phenomenon of chicken pox parties to him. I say, "Some people want their children to get chicken pox because," and pause to think of the best reason to give a doctor. "They're idiots," my father supplies.

I do not think they are idiots. But I do think they may be indulging in a variety of preindustrial nostalgia that I too find seductive. We used to live among wild things, mountain lions on the ridge and fires raging on the prairie. There were dangers, but they were part of, as Rachel Carson would say, "a natural system in perfect balance." It is difficult to imagine any type of chicken pox, with its distinctive rash described as a "dewdrop on a rose petal," as sinister. And it is hard not to suspect, when the two types of chicken pox virus are termed the *wild type* and the *vaccine virus*, that the wild type might be superior.

In 2011, a television news interview with a Nashville woman who was selling lollipops infected with chicken pox led to exposure of a "multistate ring" of parents swapping lollipops that had been licked by sick children. As a federal prosecutor was quick to point out, it is illegal to ship viruses through the mail. The ill-gotten lollipops, priced at fifty dollars apiece, were intended as a service for parents who wanted their children to develop immunity from natural infection rather than vaccination, but infectious disease experts were skeptical of the method. Though it is theoretically possible for lollipops to transmit chicken pox, the virus typically has to be inhaled to cause infection. And the varicella virus is probably too fragile to survive a trip through the mail. But lollipops could be a reliable way to transmit hardier viruses, like hep B, which can survive outside the body for at least a week. In addition to hep B, lollipops licked by sick children could potentially carry influenza, Group A strep, and staph.

Chicken pox lollipops are risky for much the same reason arm-to-arm vaccination was once dangerous—other diseases can be passed this way. A popular alternative to vaccination in the nineteenth century was variolation, the practice of purposefully infecting a person with a mild case of smallpox. Both vaccination and variolation had their dangers. Both could cause high fevers, both could result in infection, and both could pass diseases like syphilis. But variolation, which produced an illness that tended to be fatal in about 1 to 2 percent of its cases, was more dangerous than vaccination. Despite being safer, vaccination did not replace variolation immediately after Edward Jenner popularized the technique. Variolation remained popular in England, Nadja Durbach writes, in part because people preferred "what they considered 'the real thing.'"

By the time Coca-Cola was marketed under the slogan

"It's the Real Thing" in the 1940s, it no longer contained cocaine. It was not the real thing, and it had never really been the real thing. The pharmacist who developed the combination of cocaine and caffeine as a "nerve tonic" in 1886 claimed that it cured nervous disorders, headaches, and impotence. What it did was deliver an addictive stimulant in a pleasantly flavored elixir. It was an immensely popular tonic, but not because it was healthful.

The introduction of New Coke, a 1985 reformulation, did not go well despite blind taste tests that suggested people preferred it to Coca-Cola. There were lawsuits, boycotts, and public protests. That New Coke could not easily replace a product traditionally marketed on its authenticity should probably not have come as a surprise to the Coca-Cola company. We are wary of imitations, even when they offer improvements. We want the wild type, not the vaccine virus. And we would prefer for our children to have an authentic experience of chicken pox. Part of the appeal of intentional infection with chicken pox is that this form of inoculation does not resemble vaccination so much as it resembles variolation, the real thing. For nineteenth-century practitioners, variolation was a means of "taking immunity into your own hands," as Anne Moscona, a pediatric infectious disease expert, observes. It was, like our contemporary chicken pox lollipops and swine flu parties, "vigilante vaccination."

¶The concept of *Clear and Present Danger* was once used to defend mandatory vaccination in times of epidemic. And the term *conscientious objector*, now associated primarily with war, originally referred to those who refused vaccination. Britain's Compulsory Vaccination Act of 1853 required the vaccination of all infants, and was widely resisted. After later legislation allowed for resisters to be repeatedly fined, those who could not pay had their belongings seized and auctioned, or were imprisoned. In 1898, the government added a conscience clause to the act, allowing parents to apply for exemption. The clause was rather vague, requiring only that the objector "satisfy" a magistrate that her objection was a matter of conscience. This would result in thousands of cases of conscientious objection, in some places accounting for the majority of all births, as well as a debate over what exactly it meant to possess a conscience.

Before the term *conscientious objector* was written into law, it was used by vaccine resisters to distinguish themselves from negligent parents who had not bothered to vaccinate their children. The word *conscientious* was meant to signal that this was an intentional decision made by caring parents. Conscientious objectors argued that a conscience could not and should not be evaluated, and the magistrates themselves were vexed by the problem of whether or not to demand some sort of evidence to support a claim to conscience. "I don't understand the Act," one magistrate said in frustration. "I have seen you, and you have told me you have a conscientious objection; I don't know whether that is enough." The word *satisfy* was eventually removed from the conscience clause and a series of memoranda specified that an objector must hold an "honest" belief that vaccination would harm her child but that her belief need not be "reasonably founded." In debating the law, parliamentarians determined that the conscience was very difficult to define.

From the advent of the conscience clause until now, the *Oxford English Dictionary* has consistently defined conscience primarily in terms of right and wrong. "The sense of right and wrong as regards things for which one is responsible" now appears in its first definition. The next six definitions mention ethical values, justice, equity, correct judgments, scruple, knowledge, insight, and God, with feelings and heart entering into the eighth and ninth definitions, along with the notations "now rare" and "obsolete."

George Washington, a survivor of smallpox, wrestled with the question of whether or not to require inoculation for revolutionary soldiers long before vaccination became a question of conscience. In 1775, roughly a third of the Continental Army fell ill to smallpox while laying siege to Quebec. They were eventually forced to retreat in the first battlefield defeat of this country's history. The deadliest smallpox epidemic the colonies had seen was in the process of taking 100,000 lives, but smallpox was endemic in England and most of the British soldiers were immune, having survived it as children. This was before the invention of vaccination, and Washington was reluctant to subject his troops to variolation, which had known dangers and was illegal in some of the colonies. Several times, he ordered inoculation and then withdrew the order days later. Finally, with rumors in the air of a British plan to spread smallpox as a form of biological warfare, Washington definitively ordered the inoculation of all new recruits.

If we owe the existence of this nation in some part to

compulsory inoculation, we also owe some of its present character to the resistance against compulsory vaccination. Early vaccine refusers were among the first to make legal challenges to the growing reach of police power in the United States. We have them to thank for the fact that we can no longer be vaccinated at gunpoint, and perhaps also for the fact that women cannot be denied abortions. Some pivotal reproductive rights cases in the 1970s cited as their precedent *Jacobson v. Massachusetts*, a 1905 Supreme Court case in which a minister defended his refusal of vaccination on the grounds that a previous vaccination had damaged his health. But this case has also been used as a precedent for defending warrantless searches and the detainment of US citizens. The ruling in *Jacobson* was an effort to balance the interests of the collective and the power of the state against the rights of the individual. It upheld compulsory vaccination laws, but required that states offer exemptions for individuals who might be subject to injustice and oppression under those laws.

The United States has never had a federal compulsory vaccination law. In the early twentieth century some states had compulsory laws, but two-thirds of the states did not, and a couple states had laws against compulsion. In some school districts, children were—as they are now—required to be vaccinated in order to attend public school, but this requirement was often loosely enforced. A third of the school children in Greenville, Pennsylvania, for example, were granted medical exemptions from vaccination.

The only vaccine routinely recommended at that time was the smallpox vaccine, which had serious side effects and was frequently contaminated with bacteria. A new, milder strain of smallpox appeared in this country around the turn of the century and *Variola minor*, as it is now known, was killing only around 1 percent of the people who contracted it, as opposed to the 30 percent who typically died from *Variola major*. With smallpox taking fewer lives, unorganized opposition to vaccination became an antivaccination movement led by activists like Lora Little, who offered empowering advice: "Be your own doctor. Run your own machine." In some places, armed mobs drove vaccinators away. "Vaccination riots," the journalist Arthur Allen writes, "were not at all uncommon."

Long before the term *immunity* was used in the context of disease, it was used in the context of law to describe an exemption from service or duty to the state. *Immunity* came to mean freedom from disease as well as freedom from service in the late nineteenth century, after states began requiring vaccination. In a peculiar collision of meanings, the exemption from immunity made possible by the conscience clause was a kind of immunity in itself. And allowing oneself to remain vulnerable to disease remains a legal privilege today.

Dictionaries aside, what it means to have a conscience may be no more clear to us now than it was in 1898. We do recognize when it is lacking—*she has no conscience*, we say. But what exactly is missing? I put this question to my sister, who teaches ethics at a Jesuit college and is a member of the North American Kant Society. "It's tricky," she says. "In the eighteenth century, Kant wrote that we have a duty to ourselves to examine our conscience. This implies that it's not transparent, that it must be scrutinized and deciphered. Kant thought of conscience as an inner judge and used the metaphor of a courtroom to explain its operation. In the courtroom of conscience, the self is both judge and judged."

I ask her if this means our conscience emerges from thought and is a product of our minds. "It's an evolving concept," she says. "It may have once been more closely associated with the emotions, but we still say we *feel a pang of conscience*—it involves a unity of thought and feeling." Kant, she tells me, called the inner judge a "scrutinizer of hearts."

"The part that's tricky," my sister says, "is how you discern between a sense of discomfort and what your conscience is telling you." This question remains with me, and I am disturbed by the possibility that I could mistake the call of my conscience for something else. I ask a former professor of mine, a novelist who teaches the Old Testament as literature, how one recognizes one's own conscience. She looks at me sternly and says, "It's a very distinct feeling. I don't think one's conscience is easily confused with any other feeling."

"Morality can't be fully private," my sister tells me, "for many of the same reasons that a language can't be fully private. You can't be intelligible only to yourself. But thinking of the conscience as a private sense of right and wrong suggests that our collective understandings of justice can be insufficient. An individual might resist flaws in the dominant moral code and thus create the possibility for reform—there are all sorts of historical examples of this. But another way to think about the conscience is as an inner voice that keeps your actions in line with publicly defensible moral standards. It reforms you."

One of the mercies of immunity produced by vaccination is that a small number of people can forgo vaccination without putting themselves or others at greatly increased risk. But the exact number of people this might be—the threshold at which herd immunity is lost and the risk of disease rises dramatically for both the vaccinated and the unvaccinated—varies depending on the disease and the vaccine and the population in question. We know the threshold, in many cases, only after we've exceeded it. And so this puts the conscientious objector in the precarious position of potentially contributing to an epidemic. Here we may suffer what economists call moral hazard, a tendency to take unwise risks when we are protected by insurance. Our laws allow for some people to exempt themselves from vaccination, for reasons medical or religious or philosophical. But deciding for ourselves whether we ought to be among that number is indeed a matter of conscience.

In a section of *The Vaccine Book* titled "Is it your social responsibility to vaccinate your kids?" Dr. Bob asks, "Can we fault parents for putting their own child's health ahead of that of the kids around him?" This is meant to be a rhetorical question, but Dr. Bob's implied answer is not mine. In another section of the book, Dr. Bob writes of his advice to parents who fear the MMR vaccine, "I also warn them not to share their fears with their neighbors, because if too many people avoid the MMR, we'll likely see the disease increase significantly."

I do not need to consult an ethicist to determine that there is something wrong there, but my sister clarifies my discomfort. "The problem is in making a special exemption just for yourself," she says. This reminds her of a way of thinking proposed by the philosopher John Rawls: Imagine that you do not know what position you are going to hold in society—rich, poor, educated, insured, no access to health care, infant, adult, HIV positive, healthy immune system, etc.—but that you are aware of the full range of possibilities. What you would want in that situation is a policy that is going to be equally just no matter what position you end up in.

"Consider relationships of dependence," my sister suggests. "You don't own your body—that's not what we are, our bodies aren't independent. The health of our bodies always depends on choices other people are making." She falters for a moment here, and is at a loss for words, which is rare for her. "I don't even know how to talk about this," she says. "The point is there's an illusion of independence."

¶ On becoming queen in 1558, Elizabeth I spoke of inhabiting two bodies: "I am but one body naturally considered, though by His permission a body politic to govern." She drew this idea from medieval political theology, but the notion of a body politic was already ancient then. The Greeks imagined the body politic as an organism, itself alive and part of a greater cosmic organism—both the citizen and the city were bodies within bodies.

Our contemporary belief that we inhabit only one body contained entirely within the boundaries of our skin emerged from Enlightenment thinking, which celebrated the individual in both mind and body. But what defined an individual remained somewhat elusive. By the end of the Age of Enlightenment, the body of a slave was allowed to represent only three-fifths of a person. Some people remained parts of a whole while others enjoyed the novel illusion of being whole unto themselves.

In response to a 1912 definition of biological individuality as the quality of being "rendered nonfunctional if cut in half," Donna Haraway observes that this requirement of indivisibility is problematic for both worms and women. "That, of course," Haraway writes, "is why women have had so much trouble counting as individuals in modern Western discourses. Their personal, bounded individuality is compromised by their bodies' troubling talent for making other bodies, whose individuality can take precedence over their own, even while the little bodies are fully contained." One of our functions, as women, is to be divided.

When my son asks me about his belly button, I describe the near-mythological umbilical cord that once connected us. I point to my belly button and tell him that all of us were once contained within another body on which our lives depended. Even a three-year-old, who is still wholly dependent on me but already accustomed to thinking of himself as independent, finds this perplexing. Speaking from a moment just before the Enlightenment, Queen Elizabeth expressed a paradox that eludes us to this day—our bodies may belong to us, but we ourselves belong to a greater body composed of many bodies. We are, bodily, both independent and dependent.

The natural body meets the body politic in the act of vaccination, where a single needle penetrates both. The capacity of some vaccines to generate a collective immunity superior to the individual immunity produced by those same vaccines suggests that the politic has not only a body, but also an immune system capable of protecting it as a whole. Some of us assume that what is good for the body politic cannot be good for the body natural—that the interests of these bodies must be at odds. But the work of epidemiologists and immunologists and even mathematicians often suggests otherwise. All sorts of risk-benefit analyses and models of herd immunity tend to produce the conclusion that vaccination benefits the individual as well as the public. When Harvard researchers recently used game theory to build a mathematical model of vaccination behavior during an influenza epidemic, they found that even "a population of self-interested people can defeat an epidemic." No altruism is required.

Vaccines are regulated, recommended, and distributed by the state—there is a very literal relationship between government and vaccination. But there is a metaphoric relationship too. Vaccines govern the immune system, in the sense that they impose a particular order on it. British antivaccinators in the nineteenth century compared their movement to the Irish Home Rule movement, conflating the governance of a country with the governance of a body. We resist vaccination in part because we want to rule ourselves.

Attitudes toward the state easily translate into attitudes toward vaccination, in part because the body is such a ready metaphor for the nation. The state has a head, of course, and the government has arms, with which it can overreach its power. In *I Is an Other*, James Geary writes of an experiment designed to study the effects of using the body as a metaphor for the nation. Researchers invited two groups of people to read an article about US history that used bodily metaphors—the nation experienced a "growth spurt" and worked to "digest" innovations. Before reading this article, one of the groups was also asked to read an article describing airborne bacteria as harmful. Researchers found that the group of people who had read about harmful bacteria were later more likely than the people who had not to express both concern about bodily contamination and negative opinions on immigration, though the article about US history had not mentioned immigration. Without having the metaphor explicitly established for them, those people gravitated toward thinking of immigrants as bacteria, invasively contaminating the body of the nation. Where two issues are metaphorically linked, the researchers concluded, manipulating a person's attitude toward one can affect how she thinks about the other.

"If thought corrupts language," George Orwell famously suggested, "language can also corrupt thought." Stale metaphors reproduce stale thinking. Mixed metaphors confuse. And metaphors flow in two directions—

thinking about one thing in terms of another can illuminate or obscure both. If our sense of bodily vulnerability can pollute our politics, then our sense of political powerlessness must inform how we treat our bodies.

¶ In the spring following the H1N1 flu pandemic, when my son was a year old, the Deepwater Horizon oil rig exploded. Eleven workers were killed, and a well-head on the sea floor began spilling oil into the Gulf of Mexico. It spilled 210 million gallons of oil over eighty-seven days. The mothers I knew were no longer talking about the flu, but we did talk about the oil spill. None of us said this explicitly, but the spill that kept spilling seemed emblematic of everything we could not control in our children's lives.

One day that spring I called my husband in tears to tell him that we needed to get a new mattress for our son's crib. "Okay," he said carefully, understanding neither the need for the new mattress nor my tears. That morning my reading on vaccines had led me, through a meandering course, to an article about the chemicals used to plasticize plastics, which had led me to an article about the potential health hazards of plastic baby bottles, which had led me to an article about the gases released by the plastic often used to cover infant mattresses. Much of the research on this subject was preliminary, and many of the concerns were speculative. But I had read enough, by noon, to begin to wonder about my son's mattress, where he slept an average of twelve hours a night. After examining the tag on the mattress and corresponding with the manufacturer, I talked to my father, who assured me that my son was fine, given all the air circulating around him while he slept, but acknowledged that, yes, he knew of a case in which people had been sickened by car interiors made of polyvinyl chloride, the type of plastic that covered my son's mattress.

It wasn't this that brought me to tears. It was that I had already, in that first year of my child's life, discovered that some disposable diapers contained a chemical that gave him a red burning rash. And that the toothpaste I first used on his four tiny teeth, a "natural" brand, contained an additive that blistered the inside of his mouth. My son, like me, is unusually sensitive to certain chemicals, so I tried not to take this as an indication that we were swimming in danger. But after I learned, from another mother, that the FDA does not have the authority to regulate cosmetics, including shampoos and lotions for babies, in the way it regulates pharmaceuticals, I found myself paralyzed in the drugstore, staring at the ingredients of the lotion our pediatrician had recommended for my son's skin, badly chapped by the wind whipping off Lake Michigan.

At that moment, unprecedented amounts of Corexit, a chemical dispersant, were being sprayed onto the Deepwater oil spill from airplanes. Corexit was one of 62,000 chemicals grandfathered under the Toxic Substances Control Act of 1976 without any health or safety review. Oil dispersants are, like the chemicals in my son's mattress, plasticizers. But the plasticizers in the mattress become infinitesimal when compared to the 1.84 million gallons of dispersant spilled onto the spill. As the Environmental Protection Agency observed at the time, Corexit was neither the safest nor the most effective dispersant on the market—it was simply the most readily available to BP in the wake of the spill. That May, the EPA requested that a less toxic dispersant be used on the spill, but BP did not comply. While a full understanding of its toxicity is still emerging, Corexit's primary virtue seems to have been that it made the oil spill appear to disappear.

I was not comforted that the oil, in some less visible form, was still roiling through the water, killing coral and sea turtles and dolphins, endangering everything from whale sharks to sea grass. In the wake of the collapse of a deregulated financial industry, I was panicked by the spillage of a poorly regulated oil industry and the leakage of an underregulated chemical industry. "If our government," I cried to my husband, "can't keep phthalates out of my baby's bedroom and parabens out of his lotion, and 210 million gallons of crude oil and 1.84 million gallons of dispersant out of the Gulf of Mexico, for the love of God, then what is it good for?" There was a pause. "I hear you," my husband said in a voice that I recognized as the first measure in a concerted effort to contain my runaway anxiety. "Let's just get a new mattress for now," he said. "Let's start there."

In immunology, the term *regulation* refers to the strategies the body employs to avoid doing damage to itself. We feel sick when we are sick in part because our immune system is not entirely benevolent to our body. The fever that slows the growth of bacteria can, if it becomes too high, damage the body's enzymes. The inflammation that protects cells can, if allowed to persist unchecked, harm tissues. And the chemical signals essential to an immune response can, in excessive amounts, lead to organ failure. When protective impulses are unregulated, they can be as dangerous as they are necessary.

"In the fall of 1901, regulation was a controversial idea," the historian Michael Willrich writes. "A few months later, it was federal law." What happened in between was a smallpox outbreak in Camden, New Jersey, where nine children died after receiving a smallpox vaccine contaminated with tetanus. Over the next century, the production of vaccines would slowly become one of our better-regulated industries. Vaccine manufacture and testing is now overseen by the FDA and the CDC, and vaccine safety is evaluated by periodic independent reviews conducted by the Institute of Medicine. Vaccines are subject to ongoing surveillance through a national database that collects reports of side effects and a database that tracks medical records from large health care providers. But the presence of regulation resembles the absence of regulation in that neither is highly visible.

"What else is in the air that I can't see?" my son asks after I explain radio waves to him. I tell him about X-rays and microwaves. When I pause, wondering whether to mention radon and pollution, my husband begins talking about sunlight. "Explosions on the sun make tiny particles, called neutrinos," he tells our son. "These fly off the sun and travel through the atmosphere. They are so small that they pass right through our bodies without us ever feeling them. Think of that—we have little bits of the sun pouring right through our bodies all the time! We have sunshine in us!"

I am grateful for this ode to the unseen because I have just read *Silent Spring* and my mind is full of malevolent invisibles. "In this now universal contamination of the environment," Carson writes, "chemicals are the sinister and little-recognized partners of radiation in changing the very nature of the world—the very nature of its life." This may be true, but radiation also takes the form, as my husband reminds me, of sunshine.

It is both a luxury and a hazard to feel threatened by the invisible. In Chicago, where 677 children were shot the year after my son was born, I still somehow manage to find myself more captivated by less tangible threats. While two-year-olds take bullets in other parts of the city, I worry over the danger embedded in the paint that chips off my child's toys and the walls around him. I fear that it is woven into the clothes he wears, that it is in the air he breathes, in the water he drinks, and in the compromised food I feed him.

If we understand ourselves as living in a world of unseen evils, the immune system, that largely conceptual entity devoted to protecting us from invisible threats, will inevitably take on an inflated importance and a distorted function. "The imperilled 'immune system,'" the physician Michael Fitzpatrick observes, "is a metaphor for the prevailing sense of the vulnerability of the human individual in a hostile world."

The term *immune system*, he notes, was probably a metaphor from its very introduction. In a medical context, the word *system* traditionally referred to a collection of organs or tissue, but the immunologists who first adopted it were using it in a broader sense. "Why was the term *immune system* accepted so widely and so rapidly?" asks the historian of immunology Anne-Marie Moulin. The answer, she suggests, resides in its "linguistic versatility," the ability of the term to contain many concepts and multiple understandings. It entered the mainstream just a few years after its introduction to science, spilling into the popular usage of the 1970s. "Though the term was borrowed from the science of immunology," Fitzpatrick writes, "its new meaning was filled out with ideas derived from influential contemporary trends, notably environmentalism, alternative health and New Age mysticism."

The immune system also gathered significance from the emergence of systems theory in the natural and social sciences. Systems theory, the anthropologist Emily Martin observes, has become a pervasive model for how we think about both our environment and our bodies. Where the machine with its distinct components was once the most available metaphor for the body, we now tend to think of the body as a complex system—a sensitive, nonlinear field with elaborate regulatory mechanisms.

"What are some of the possible or likely consequences of thinking of the body as a complex system?" Martin asks. "The first consequence might be described as the paradox of feeling responsible for everything and powerless at the same time, a kind of empowered powerlessness." If one feels at least partly responsible for one's own health, she explains, but understands one's body as a complex system linked to other complex systems, including the community and the environment, the task of controlling all the factors that might affect one's health becomes overwhelming.

Feeling responsible for everything and powerless at the same time is also a good description, I think, of the emotional state induced by US citizenship. Our representative democracy endows us with empowered powerlessness. This is a problem of governance, but it is also, as Rachel Carson would suggest, something else. "For each of us, as for the robin in Michigan or the salmon in the Miramichi," she writes, "this is a problem of ecology, of interrelationships, of interdependence."

¶ Everyone who is born holds dual citizenship, in the kingdom of the well and in the kingdom of the sick," Susan Sontag wrote in her introduction to *Illness as Metaphor*. "Although we all prefer to use only the good passport, sooner or later each of us is obliged, at least for a spell, to identify ourselves as citizens of that other place."

Sontag wrote these words while being treated for cancer, not knowing how much time she had left to live. She wrote, she later explained, to "calm the imagination." Those of us who have lived most of our lives in the kingdom of the well may find our imaginations already placid. Not all of us think of health as a transient state that we may be exiled from without warning. Some prefer to assume health as an identity. *I am healthy*, we tell each other, meaning that we eat certain foods and avoid others, that we exercise and do not smoke. Health, it is implied, is the reward for living the way we live, and lifestyle is its own variety of immunity.

When health becomes an identity, sickness becomes not something that happens to you, but who you are. Your style of life, I gleaned from the way the word *lifestyle* was used in junior high school health class, is either clean or dirty, safe or unsafe, free of disease or prone to disease. Health class in my school was devoted largely to AIDS education, and this was late enough in the epidemic that we were repeatedly reminded—while being informed on all the ways the disease could be transmitted —that AIDS was not spread through casual contact. To encourage our empathy for the infected, we were shown a documentary about a hemophiliac boy who contracted HIV through a blood transfusion. He had not engaged in any of the risky behavior we had been warned against in class, and the intended message was

141

that innocent victims of this disease did in fact exist. The unspoken corollary was that other people with HIV were to blame for their infection.

My generation came of age in the shadow of the AIDS epidemic, and it seems to have left us believing not that we are all vulnerable to disease, but that it is possible to avoid disease by living a cautious life and limiting our contact with others. "Cancerphobia taught us the fear of a polluting environment," Sontag writes, and "now we have the fear of polluting people that AIDS anxiety inevitably communicates. Fear of the Communion cup, fear of surgery: fear of contaminated blood, whether Christ's blood or your neighbor's. Life—blood, sexual fluids—is itself the bearer of contamination."

The anxieties generated by the AIDS epidemic have bled into our attitudes toward vaccination. Needles, as we learned from AIDS, can spread disease. The needle itself has become "dirty." AIDS reveals that our immune systems are vulnerable to sabotage and can be permanently disabled. Vaccines, which engage the immune system, are now suspect as potential saboteurs, capable, we fear, of producing autoimmune diseases or overwhelming a child's immune system. This fear of an immune system being "overwhelmed" can itself be traced back to AIDS—the HIV virus, as I learned in health class, hides in our T cells, quietly proliferating until it releases an explosion of copies of itself that overwhelms our system. And then there is the unsettling presence, however remote or conceptual, of other people's blood and bodies in vaccines themselves. Robbed of their context, some of the components involved in vaccine production—human albumin, protein fragments from human cells, residual DNA—suggest that debris from other bodies is being injected into us.

AIDS education taught us the importance of protecting our bodies from contact with other bodies, and this seems to have bred another kind of insularity, a preoccupation with the integrity of the individual immune system. Building, boosting, and supplementing one's personal immune system is a kind of cultural obsession of the moment. I know mothers who believe this is a viable substitute for vaccination, and who understand themselves as raising children with superior immune systems. But children with superior immune systems can still pass disease. Pertussis, like polio and Hib disease and HIV, can be carried without symptoms. When I asked a friend how she would feel if her child contracted an infectious disease and did not suffer from it but passed it to someone more vulnerable who would suffer, she looked at me in surprise. She had not, she told me, considered that possibility.

"Is the immune system at the heart of a new incarnation of social Darwinism that allows people of different 'quality' to be distinguished from each other?" asks the anthropologist Emily Martin. She believes the answer may be yes. Some of the people in her study expressed what she calls "immune machismo," saying, for instance, that their immune systems "kick ass." One person suggested, in Martin's words, that "people without a good living standard need vaccines, whereas vaccines would only clog up the more refined systems of middle-class or upper-class people." Even assuming that certain immune systems do kick ass, the problem remains that vaccination is most dangerous, in many cases, for people with compromised immune systems. Those of us with impaired immunity depend on people with more functional immune systems to carry immunity and protect us from disease.

"AIDS is everyone's problem," the vice president of the Red Cross announced in 1987, though media coverage, the journalist Richard Goldstein observed, positioned the average American as a witness to the epidemic, safe from infection. I have found myself so positioned, invited to regard AIDS as a problem that belongs to gay men and Africa. Disease happens to other people, this thinking implies, people who are not good or clean. That this attitude extends beyond AIDS is evident in the indignation expressed over the vaccination of newborn infants against hep B, another disease passed through blood. The hep B vaccine is often used to illustrate the absurdity of a public health system that would vaccinate a newborn baby against a sexually transmitted disease.

"Why target two and a half million innocent newborns and children?" Barbara Loe Fisher asks of the hep B vaccine. The implication behind the word *innocent* is that only those who are not innocent need protection from disease. All of us who grew up during the AIDS epidemic were exposed to the idea that AIDS was a punishment for homosexuality, promiscuity, and addiction. But if disease is a punishment for anything, it is only a punishment for being alive.

When I was a child, I asked my father what causes cancer and he paused for a long moment before saying, "Life. Life causes cancer." I took this as an artful dodge until I read Siddhartha Mukherjee's history of cancer, in which he argues not only that life causes cancer but that cancer is us. "Down to their innate molecular core," Mukherjee writes, "cancer cells are hyperactive, survival-endowed, scrappy, fecund, inventive copies of ourselves." And this, he notes, "is not a metaphor."

¶ I gave my son a lavishly illustrated edition of *Alice's Adventures in Wonderland* for his fourth birthday, and it did not take very long for me to realize that this was a gift for me, not him. As Alice engaged in repartee with a dodo early in the book, my son became bored. Alice's bewilderment and disorientation, which I had anticipated might speak to my son's experience of being a child in an adult's world, spoke instead to my own experience navigating the world of information. Being lost in Wonderland is what it feels like to learn about an unfamiliar subject, and research is inevitably a rabbit hole. I fell down it, in my investigation of immunization, and fell and fell, finding that it was much deeper than I anticipated. Like Alice, I fell past shelves full of books, more than I could ever read. Like Alice, I arrived at locked doors. "Drink me," I was commanded by one source. "Eat me," I was told by another. They had opposite effects—I grew and shrank, I believed and did not believe. I cried and then found myself swimming in my own tears.

Early in my research, I read an article about three cases of potential vaccine injury that had been winding their way through the courts for the past seven years and had finally been decided. These three cases had been selected as the strongest of more than five thousand similar cases brought to a special division of the US Court of Federal Claims popularly known as "Vaccine Court" and were serving as test cases to determine whether autism could be considered a vaccine injury.

The burden of proof in Vaccine Court is relatively light, and cases are heard by specially appointed attorneys who use "more probable than not" as their guideline for judgment, or as one of these special masters put it, "fifty percent plus a feather." Even so, the evidence that vaccination led to autism was insufficient in all three test cases. And the evidence against it was, as one special master would note, "overwhelming." In her decision on *Colten Snyder vs. HHS*, Special Master Denise Vowell wrote, "To conclude that Colten's condition was the result of his MMR vaccine, an objective observer would have to emulate Lewis Carroll's White Queen and be able to believe six impossible (or at least highly improbable) things before breakfast."

The problem, of course, is that believing highly improbable things is something we all do before breakfast. What makes science thrilling is the suggestion that improbable things are indeed possible. The idea, for instance, that pus from a sick cow can be scraped into a wound on a person and make that person immune to a deadly disease is almost as hard to believe now as it was in 1796. When we engage with science, we are in Wonderland. This seems as true for scientists as it is for lay people. But the difference for those of us who are not scientists is that, as with other news, what gets reported back to us most often from the land of science is that which supports our existing fears.

In the years since I became pregnant with my son, I have read about studies suggesting a link between autism and a family's proximity to a freeway, the mother's use of antidepressants, the father's age at conception, and the mother's infection with influenza during pregnancy. But none of these have enjoyed the kind of press devoted to one small, inconclusive study that suggested a link between vaccination and autism. "We live in a media culture," the writer Maria Popova observes, "that warps seeds of scientific understanding into sensationalist, definitive headlines about the gene for obesity or language or homosexuality and maps where, precisely, love or fear or the appreciation of Jane Austen is located in the brain—even though we know that it isn't the clinging to answers but the embracing of ignorance that drives science."

Overwhelmed by information in my research on vaccination, I began to notice that information itself is overwhelmed at times. While searching for the source of a rumor that the H1N1 vaccine contained squalene, I found dozens of websites and blogs with relevant articles, but they were all the same article, "Squalene: The Swine Flu Vaccine's Dirty Little Secret Exposed," written by the physician Joseph Mercola and originally self-published on his website. The reproductions of Mercola's article that proliferated across the web early in the pandemic were then, and still remain, uncorrected. But by the time I traced them to the version on his website in the fall of 2009, the original article already included a correction in the header clarifying that none of the H1N1 vaccines distributed in the United States contained squalene. This was not a minor point of correction, but the article had gone viral before being corrected. Like a virus, it had replicated itself repeatedly, overwhelming more credible information about the vaccine.

For centuries before the word *virus* was first used to describe a specific type of microorganism, it was used more generally for anything that spread disease—pus, air, even paper. Now a bit of computer code or the content of a website can be viral. But, as with the kind of virus that infects humans, this content cannot reproduce without hosts.

Misinformation that finds a host enjoys a kind of immortality on the Internet, where it becomes undead.

When I asked some other mothers to share with me the information on which they had based their vaccination decisions, one of the first articles I was sent was "Deadly Immunity" by Robert F. Kennedy Jr. It had been published in *Rolling Stone* magazine and online by *Salon*, where it had accumulated, by the time I read it, five significant factual corrections. A year later, *Salon* retracted it entirely. This unusual decision, the editor explained, was made in part because the story was flawed not just in its facts, but also in its logic, which was more difficult to correct. A former editor was critical of the retraction, noting that removing the article from *Salon*'s site did not make it unavailable—it is hosted on a number of other sites—but erased the only version of the article that had been corrected.

Science is, as scientists like to say, "self-correcting," meaning that errors in preliminary studies are, ideally, revealed by subsequent studies. One of the primary principles of the scientific method is that the results of a study must be reproducible. Until the results of a small study are duplicated by a larger study, they are little more than a suggestion for further research. Most studies are not incredibly meaningful on their own, but gain or lose meaning from the work that has been done around them. And, as the medical researcher John Ioannidis has observed, "most published research findings are false." The reasons for this are many, and include bias, study size, study design, and the very questions the researcher is asking. This does not mean that published research should be disregarded, but that, as Ioannidis concludes, "What matters is the totality of the evidence."

Thinking of our knowledge as a body suggests the harm that can be done when one part of that body is torn from its context. Quite a bit of this sort of dismemberment goes on in discussions about vaccination, where individual studies are often used to support positions or ideas that are not supported by the body as a whole. "Any science may be likened to a river," proposes the biologist Carl Swanson. "It has its obscure and unpretentious beginning; its quiet stretches as well as its rapids, its periods of drought as well as of fullness. It gathers momentum with the work of many investigators and as it is fed by other streams of thought; it is deepened and broadened by the concepts and generalizations that are gradually evolved."

When one is investigating scientific evidence, one must consider the full body of information, or survey the full body of water. And if the body is large, this becomes an impossible task for one single person. A committee of eighteen medical experts took two years, for instance, to examine 12,000 peer-reviewed articles in order to prepare their 2011 report on vaccine side effects for the Institute of Medicine. The committee included a specialist in research methods, an expert on autoimmune disorders, a medical ethicist, an authority on childhood immune responses, a child neurologist, and a researcher dedicated to studying brain development. In addition to confirming the relative safety of vaccines, their report illustrated the kind of collaboration required to navigate the information now available to us. We do not know alone.

Dracula was published in 1897, at a time when education reform in Britain had led to unprecedented literacy rates. Information was moving in new ways, reaching people it had not reached before. This was also a time in which new technologies were rapidly emerging and

149

changing the way people lived. A time, in other words, not unlike our own.

Many new inventions of the day are featured in *Dracula*, including the typewriter. The setting of the novel is "nineteenth century up-to-date with a vengeance," as one of the characters observes, before adding ominously, "And yet, unless my senses deceive me, the old centuries had, and have, powers of their own which mere 'modernity' cannot kill." The heroine of *Dracula* is a working woman who types her own diary and transcribes a number of other documents that become, collectively, the novel. The extent to which its plot depends on the typewriter suggests that this book is, in part, about technologies for reproducing information. Bram Stoker seems optimistic about these technologies, in that they contribute to the triumph of good over evil. But anxieties over the uncertainties of modern life drive the plot of the novel and, as an 1897 review noted, the vampire is ultimately slain in a medieval fashion—an Englishman beheads him while an American plunges a Bowie knife through his heart.

Dracula has no single narrator. The story unfolds through a collection of diary entries, letters, and newspaper articles. Each of these documents records the observations of a person who has witnessed something of Dracula's doings, and only by putting these observations together does enough evidence emerge for the central characters to conclude that they are dealing with a vampire. Very early in the book a character notes in his diary, after meeting Dracula for the first time, that his hand is cold, "more like the hand of a dead than a living man," but Dracula will not be exposed as undead until much later. The reader, having access to all the documents, inevitably understands what is going on long before anyone else does.

The vampire hunters refer to their growing collection of documents often, as if their observations would not exist without them. "One can see the insistence throughout the text," the literary critic Allan Johnson writes, "of the fundamental value of recorded, empirical knowledge in the fight against the mysterious unknown." Dracula is the unknown, as much as he is disease. The novel asks *How do we know what we know?* This is a question intended to unsettle the reader, and over a century later it is still an unsettling question.

Just before he leaves London, Count Dracula takes revenge on his pursuers by throwing their original documents, the diaries and letters and recordings they have been keeping of their observations, into a fire. All that is left is a typewritten copy of those documents, which we are to understand is the book we have just read. Because it is a copy and not an original, it is, as one character observes in his final note at the end of the book, not to be believed. "We could hardly ask anyone, even did we wish to," he writes, "to accept these as proofs of so wild a story."

Knowledge is, by its nature, always incomplete. "A scientist is never certain," the scientist Richard Feynman reminds us. And neither, the poet John Keats would argue, is a poet. "Negative capability" was his term for the ability to dwell in uncertainty. My mother, a poet, has been instilling this ability in me since I was a child. "You have to erase yourself," she says, meaning abandon what I think I know. Or "live the questions," as Rainer Maria Rilke writes in his *Letters to a Young Poet*. This, my mother reminds me, is as essential to mothering as it is to poetry—we must live the questions our children raise for us.

¶ Shortly after he turned four, my son slept in my arms like a heavy newborn baby while a doctor impressed on me that his allergies, which now included some food allergies, could pose a serious threat to his health. My observations, in part, had brought us to this diagnosis, but I doubted both myself and the doctor as I looked down at my son, who appeared perfectly unthreatened in his sleep. After the doctor left the room, a nurse demonstrated the EpiPen I would need to use if my son ever had a life-threatening reaction to nuts. "I know," she said when she saw tears well up in my eyes while she pretended to jab herself forcefully in the thigh with the syringe. "I hope you never have to do this." Later I would dutifully read all the information the doctor had given me, while still maintaining the secret belief that none of it was true and that food could not hurt my child.

In the lists upon lists of things my son was advised by the doctor to avoid, one item in particular caught my attention—the seasonal flu shot. Children with egg allergies can react to this particular vaccine, which is grown in eggs. My son had already been vaccinated against the flu, just as he had already eaten many eggs, but I could see the irony in the possibility that a vaccine posed him special danger. Thinking with the logic of a Greek myth, I wondered if my interest in immunity had somehow invited immune dysfunction for him. Maybe I had given him, like poor Icarus, fragile wings.

I did not admit this fear to the doctor, but I did ask her what I had done to cause these allergies. I hoped to reverse the damage, or at least stem it. The possibility that I was not to blame did not initially occur to me. The doctor, herself a mother, spent some time assuring me that although the origin of allergies is mysterious, there was probably nothing I could have done differently. I myself have allergies, as does my husband, so if I was to blame, she suggested, it was only for carrying the genetic material I carry. This did not satisfy me. Neither did anything I went on to learn about allergies, about which we seem to know very little.

There is a passage in Daniel Defoe's *A Journal of the Plague Year* in which his narrator wonders how the disease finds its victims. He does not believe, as others do, that it is simply a "Stroke from Heaven." He is certain that it is passed from one person to another, "Spread by Infection, that is to say, by some certain Steams, or Fumes, which the Physicians call *Effluvia*, by the Breath, or by the Sweat, or by the Stench of the Sores of the sick Persons, or some other way, perhaps, beyond even the Reach of the Physicians themselves…" Indeed, it would be over 150 years before physicians would know that the plague is passed by fleas.

As the plague spreads, Defoe's narrator has an understanding that contagion is at work, and some inkling of germ theory, but he rejects that theory. The idea of "invisible Creatures, who enter into the Body with the Breath, or even at the Pores with the Air, and there generate, or emit most acute Poisons" strikes him as unlikely. He has heard that if a person with the plague breathes on a piece of glass, "there might living Creatures be seen by microscope of strange monstrous and frightful Shapes, such as Dragons, Snakes, Serpents, and Devils, horrible to behold." But this, he writes, "I very much question the Truth of." Faced with the plague and unable to make sense of his own observations, the narrator is left to reckon with improbable theories and pure speculation. Several hundred years later, I find his predicament eerily familiar.

Bubonic plague still exists, but it has ceased to be the Plague. The afflictions that take the most lives worldwide are now heart disease, stroke, respiratory infections, and AIDS, which is the only one of these that tends to be characterized as a plague. The number of lives a disease claims, as Susan Sontag observes, is not what makes it a plague. In order to be promoted to plague, a disease must be particularly feared or dreaded. I have lived through the emergence of a number of well-publicized diseases, but I never felt threatened by Ebola, or SARS, or West Nile virus, or H1N1. When my son was an infant, I feared autism, which seemed to be spreading like a plague, particularly among boys. And when he developed allergies, one after another, I began to feel dread. Perhaps the final qualification for what constitutes a plague is its proximity to your own life.

"Can you imagine," I ask a friend while reading *A Journal of the Plague Year*, "seeing people all around you dying from a disease and not knowing what is causing it, or how it is passed, or who will be next?" Even as I say this, it occurs to me that my friend lived in San Francisco at the height of the AIDS epidemic, and saw nearly everyone he knew die of a disease about which almost nothing was known. San Francisco in 1989, he reminds me, was not entirely unlike London in 1665.

Later, perhaps because I am still reckoning with the strangeness of how both near and far the plague of London feels to my own time and place, I ask the same question again. "Can you imagine?" I ask my father. By his silence I understand that he can. My father sees the sick every day—a plague is endlessly unfolding before him. "We don't have bodies falling out of windows," I say to him hopefully. "We aren't digging mass graves."

"Yes," he says, "but we're seeding a bomb." He is referring to antibiotic-resistant bacteria. The overuse of antibiotics has led to strains of bacteria that are difficult to rid from the body. One, *C. difficile*, is even named for its difficulty. In the case of *C. difficile*, over 90 percent of infections occur following a course of antibiotics. An alarming number of the patients he sees in the hospital, my father tells me, are infected with resistant bacteria.

The persistence of resistant bacteria and the emergence of novel diseases are among the top public health threats of the twenty-first century. One of these threats comes from within and is the result of our modern practices. The other comes from without and cannot be anticipated by our medicine. Both speak to our most basic fears. But novel diseases, in their capacity to serve as metaphors for foreign others and anxieties about the future, tend to generate better copy. As I write, two new diseases have been making headlines. One is an avian influenza that emerged in China, the other is a novel corona virus that was first detected in Saudi Arabia. The latter, which is the most threatening new disease of the moment, has been given the unfortunate name Middle East respiratory syndrome.

In the past century there have been three major influenza pandemics, including the 1918 Spanish flu pandemic, which killed more people than the First World War. That pandemic proved particularly deadly for young adults with strong immune systems, as it caused an overwhelming immune response. In 2004, the director of the WHO announced that another major pandemic is inevitable. "It's not a matter of if, but when," a bioethicist friend tells me. With this probability in the air, novel influenza outbreaks are often accompanied by a flurry of media attention, some of which tips into fearmongering. But even when influenza is made foreign or animal with a new name, like Chinese bird flu or swine flu, we do not seem eager to imagine it as a plague. Influenza is too common to evoke our fear of the unknown. It is not exotic or remote enough to trigger our fear of alien others. It is not disfiguring enough to threaten our sense of self. It is not spread in a way that inspires moral repulsion or the threat of punishment. Influenza does not serve, in other words, as a very good metaphor for other fears—it has to be frightening simply for what it is.

The pediatrician Paul Offit mentioned to me, during an interview about his work, that he had recently seen two children hospitalized with influenza. Both had been immunized against everything on the childhood schedule except the flu, and both ended up on heart and lung machines. One lived, and the other died. "And then the next day, when someone comes into your office and says, 'I don't want to get that vaccine,' you're supposed to respect that decision?" Offit asked me. "You can respect the fear. The fear of vaccines is understandable. But you can't respect the decision—it's an unnecessary risk."

The fact that the 2009 H1N1 influenza pandemic did not take more lives is sometimes cast, oddly, as a public health failure. "When all was said and done," Dr. Bob writes, "the hype and fear around the H1N1 flu turned out to be unwarranted." The pandemic was not as bad as it could have been, but it was not inconsequential. Somewhere between 150,000 and 575,000 people died from H1N1, over half in Southeast Asia and Africa, where public health measures were scarce. Autopsies suggest that many of the previously healthy people who died of the flu were killed by their immune response—they drowned in their own lung fluid.

The complaint that preventive measures against the flu were out of proportion to the threat strikes me as better applied to our military action in Iraq than to our response to an unpredictable virus. Vaccinating in advance of the flu, critics suggest, was a foolish preemptive strike. But preemption in war has different effects than preemption in health care—rather than generating ongoing conflict, like our preemptive strike against Iraq, preventive health care can make further health care unnecessary. Either way, prevention, of war as well as disease, is not our strong point. "The idea of preventive medicine is faintly un-American," the *Chicago Tribune* noted in 1975. "It means, first, recognizing that the enemy is us."

In 2011, studies of an H1N1 vaccine used only in Europe revealed that it caused an increased incidence of narcolepsy in Finland and Sweden. Initial reports suggest that the vaccine triggered narcolepsy in about 1 out of every 12,000 teenagers vaccinated in Finland, and about 1 out of 33,000 in Sweden. Research is ongoing and there is more to know, particularly how exactly the vaccine may have contributed to narcolepsy in that particular age group and population, but the incident has already been used to confirm existing fears that we are our own enemy. A problem with a vaccine is not evidence of the inevitable shortcomings of medicine, but evidence that we are, indeed, going to destroy ourselves.

"Apocalypse," Sontag writes, "is now a long-running serial: not 'Apocalypse Now' but 'Apocalypse From Now On.' Apocalypse has become an event that is happening and not happening." In this era of uncertain apocalypse, my father has taken to reading the Stoics, which is not an entirely surprising interest for an oncologist. What he is drawn to in their philosophy, he tells me, is the idea that you cannot control what happens to you, but you can control how you feel about it. Or, as Jean-Paul Sartre put it, "Freedom is what you do with what's been done to you."

What has been done to us seems to be, among other things, that we have been made fearful. What will we do with our fear? This strikes me as a central question of both citizenship and motherhood. As mothers, we must somehow square our power with our powerlessness. We can protect our children to some extent. But we cannot make them invulnerable any more than we can make ourselves invulnerable. "Life," as Donna Haraway writes, "is a window of vulnerability."

¶ Dracula's first victim when he arrives in England is a beautiful young woman who is found weak and pale each morning but is kept alive through a series of blood transfusions. Luckily, she has three men in love with her, all eager to give their blood. One of them writes in his diary, "No man knows till he experiences it, what it is to feel his own life-blood drawn away into the veins of the woman he loves." Dracula has a taste for good-looking women, but he does not, so far as we know, feel love. Bram Stoker's Dracula did not become a vampire to spend immortality searching for his one true love, as Francis Ford Coppola's adaptation suggests. He was always heartless, even in his mortal incarnation as Vlad the Impaler. Dracula, after all, is not a person so much as he is the embodiment of disease. And the vampire hunters who pursue him are not people so much as they are metaphors for the best impulses of medicine. Vampires take blood, and vampire hunters give blood.

As I wait with my arm outstretched to give blood, I consider this distinction. My son, who has taken to wearing a cape, likes to talk about bad guys and good guys, despite my insistence that most people are both. We are both vampires and vampire hunters, caped and uncaped. I think of Stephen King's daughter, Naomi King, who once explained that while she does not care for horror as a genre she does care about theological questions of how we make friends with our monsters. "If we demonize other people," she said, "and create monsters out of each other and act monstrous—and we all have that capacity—then how do we not become monsters ourselves?"

"Want some blood?" my son recently asked me, and held the battery terminals of a defunct smoke detector against my arm in a mock transfusion. When the operation was complete, he said proudly, "Now you don't have to eat." He thinks I am a vampire. And I am, in ways. I am here giving blood as an antidote to my own vampirism. I am also giving to repay the loan I was given by some other anonymous donor. I try to imagine that donor now as I look at the people in the chairs across from me—a muscular man studying flash cards and a middle-aged woman reading a novel and a man in a business suit looking at his phone. They are the same people I might see waiting for the train, but here they are bathed in an aura of altruism.

The reasons people give blood cannot be explained by personal gain, that much we know. This does not mean that nobody has anything to gain by giving blood. In quite a few countries, including the United States, it is common practice to offer "incentives" for blood donation. In 2008, the Red Cross ran a blood drive themed "Give a Little, Buy a Lot," in which donors had a chance to win a gift card worth $1,000. *Give a Little, Buy a Lot* would also seem to be the theme of contemporary American life, and the spirit of our high holidays. But there is some research by economists suggesting that incentives can actually discourage blood donation. Offering incentives for giving, one study concluded, can insult people who want to give just for the sake of giving.

When the needles are inserted into the people across from me, I notice each of their faces twist, for just an instant, into a grimace. I dread giving blood, and because I have been sitting here imagining these others as more willing to give than myself, it is surprising to see this look flash across their faces. As the nurse pushes the needle into my arm, I feel my face make the same expression. *I, too, dislike it*, I think. I recall the character in *Dracula* who, after experiencing something like sexual ecstasy while giving blood to the woman he loves, notes in his diary that "the draining away of one's blood, no matter how willingly it be given, is a terrible feeling."

A nurse has reclined the chair of the muscular man across from me because he is feeling faint. With my donation complete and feeling a bit faint myself, I sit at the table piled with cookies and close my eyes for a moment. Two young men, barely old enough to meet the requirement that one must be eighteen to give blood, sit down next to me and one asks the other why he is giving. "They keep calling me," the other replies. "They say I have some special kind of blood that everybody needs." The first man asks what type that is. "O negative."

I open my eyes then and see that the young man who shares my blood type has dark skin. Blood types may follow patterns of ancient ancestry, but they do not obey our racial distinctions, of course. The blood type O negative is most common among the indigenous people of Central and South America and among Australian Aborigines, though it is also somewhat common in people from Western Europe and parts of Africa. We are an extended family.

"People are storing their own blood, for future use," Susan Sontag lamented in 1989. "The model of altruistic behavior in our society, giving blood anonymously, has been compromised, since no one can be sure about anonymous blood received. Not only does AIDS have the unhappy effect of reinforcing American moralism about sex; it further strengthens the culture of self-interest, which is much of what is usually praised as 'individualism.' Self-interest now receives an added boost as simple medical prudence."

161

Simple medical prudence has historically intersected with some ugly attitudes. During the Black Death that killed more than half the population of Europe in the fourteenth century, rioters burned Jews alive under the auspices of public health. Hundreds of Jewish communities were destroyed in response to accounts of an imagined conspiracy against Christians. These accounts were extracted from Jews who confessed under torture to spreading the plague by poisoning wells. Bram Stoker's rendering of Count Dracula, with a prominent nose and piles of gold and vague origins in Eastern Europe, suggests that he is intended to be read as a Jew. To make that explicit, Bela Lugosi's Dracula wore a Star of David.

In the opening chapters of Stoker's *Dracula*, the count has recently purchased property in London. The young lawyer who travels to Transylvania to finalize the real estate transaction finds that Dracula is interested in perfecting his English. The library of his castle is full of books on British history and geography, and Dracula is even reading British train schedules. He seems to be planning a permanent relocation. And so the novel, as it unfolds, appeals to fears of immigration as well as contagion.

Avoidance of outsiders, of immigrants, of people missing limbs, or people with marks on their faces is an ancient tactic for disease prevention. And this has fed, no doubt, the long standing belief that disease is a product of those we define as others. Syphilis, Sontag writes, "was the 'French Pox' to the English, *morbus Germanicus* to the Parisians, the Naples sickness to the Florentines, the Chinese disease to the Japanese." This conflation of otherness with disease is, some would suggest, written onto our brains. Evolutionary psychologists describe a "behavioral immune system" that causes us to be highly sensitive to physical differences or unusual behavior in other people.

Our behavioral immune system can easily be triggered by people who pose us no risk. We may practice disease aversion around people with physical differences like obesity or disability, or we may practice it around groups with distinct cultural practices, like immigrants or gay men. As the American Medical Association recently observed, the ban on gay men giving blood, which was instituted in 1983, seems to have outlasted its medical prudence and is now merely discriminatory. Our tendency toward prejudice can increase whenever we feel particularly vulnerable or threatened by disease. One study has suggested, for instance, that pregnant women become more xenophobic in the early stages of pregnancy. The more vulnerable we feel, sadly, the more small-minded we become.

In the fall of 2009, at the height of the H1N1 flu pandemic, a group of researchers began testing their hypothesis that people who feel protected from disease might also be protected from feeling prejudice. The study looked at two groups of people, one vaccinated against the flu and the other not vaccinated. After both groups were asked to read an article exaggerating the threat posed by the flu, the vaccinated people expressed less prejudice against immigrants than the unvaccinated people.

The researchers went on to study how manipulating a vaccinated person's understanding of vaccination might affect that person's tendency toward prejudice. They found that framing vaccination in terms of contamination, as in "the seasonal flu vaccine involves injecting people with the seasonal flu virus," can increase prejudice in people who are concerned about disease, while framing it in terms of protection, as in "the seasonal flu vaccine protects people from the seasonal flu virus," does not. Both statements are true, incidentally, but they trigger different attitudes. After conducting one more study involving hand washing, the researchers reported a consistent pattern in their findings across all three studies: "Treatments for physical diseases, such as the flu, can also be used to treat social maladies, such as prejudice."

I have doubts that we can vaccinate away our prejudices, or wash our hands of them. There will always be diseases against which we cannot protect ourselves, and those diseases will always tempt us to project our fears onto other people. But I still believe there are reasons to vaccinate that transcend medicine.

¶ Narcissus, in Greek mythology, was a handsome hunter who was not moved by the love of others. The nymph Echo pursued him through the woods, calling out to him, but he rejected her advances and she wandered alone until she became only a faint voice calling to other voices in the woods. The god of revenge punished Narcissus for this cruelty by drawing him to a pool of water, where he fell in love with his own reflection. Heartsick for himself, Narcissus died gazing into the pool.

A painting of Narcissus at the pool was the cover illustration for a 2002 edition of *Science* dedicated to "Reflections on Self: Immunity and Beyond." The concept of self is fundamental to the science of immunity, and the dominant thinking in immunology is that the immune system must discriminate between self and nonself, and then eliminate or contain the nonself within protective barriers. The introductory article in *Science* begins with the myth of Narcissus as a metaphor for the importance of being able to recognize one's self. But a more obvious reading of that myth is as a cautionary tale for what can happen when one becomes overly absorbed with one's self and fails to appreciate the beauty of others.

I find the term *nonself* both perplexing and amusingly non-committal. Just as *undead* seems to mean something between living and dead, *nonself* seems to mean something between self and other. Nonself, I suppose, is an apt description of the human condition. In terms of sheer numbers of cells, our bodies contain more other than self. An alien looking down at us from outer space, an immunologist quips, might reasonably believe that we are just transportation for microbes. But we are using them as much as they are using us. They aid our digestion and help us synthesize vitamins and prevent the growth of harmful bacteria. Considering how dependent we are on them, it seems only right that we do not regard them as "others," exactly.

Pregnancy, which confounded my personal understanding of the distinction between self and nonself, also puzzled immunologists for quite some time. Why a woman's body would "tolerate" the nonself within her was a persistent mystery for much of the twentieth century. A whimsical theory emerged in the 1980s that sex itself served as an inoculation, with the injection of sperm into the uterus effectively vaccinating a woman against the threat posed by the fetus. That theory was abandoned in favor of the idea that the fetus does not actually share the mother's body, but is simply housed there within protective barriers, like the microbes that are housed in her gut and lungs. A further refinement of this thinking suggests that both those microbes and the fetus are given safe haven because the body does not see them as dangerous.

The possibility that patterns or signals associated with danger are what trigger an immune response was proposed by the immunologist Polly Matzinger in 1994. The Danger Model, as Matzinger writes, is "based on the idea that the immune system is more concerned with entities that do damage than with those that are foreign." The task of the immune system, following this thinking, is not to detect nonself, but to detect danger. Self can be dangerous, as immunologists have observed, and nonself can be harmless.

"It isn't really insurrectionary—it's just a different way of looking at things," Matzinger told the *New York Times* of her theory. "Imagine a community in which the police accept anyone they met during elementary school and kill any new migrant. That's the Self/Nonself Model. In the Danger Model, tourists and immigrants are accepted, until they start breaking windows. Only then, do the police move to eliminate them. In fact, it doesn't matter if the window breaker is a foreigner or a member of the community. That kind of behavior is considered unacceptable, and the destructive individual is removed." The immune system does not work alone in its efforts to detect danger, Matzinger proposes, but is in constant communication with a network of body tissues—what she calls an "extended family." If we can better understand the relationships within this family, and how the body talks with its multiple selves, then, Matzinger suggests, "we may regain a renewed sense of the self that we have lost."

The womb is sterile, and so birth is the original inoculation. Passing through the birth canal, an infant is introduced to the microbes that will inhabit that infant's skin and mouth and lungs and gut for years to come. From birth onward, our bodies are a shared space. And a failure to acquire all the necessary microbes early in life can have lasting consequences for a child's health. We are not just "tolerating" the nonself within us, we are dependent on it and protected by it. This would seem to be true, too, of the other nonselves we live among.

Diversity is essential to the health of any ecosystem. But the language we use around racial diversity, particularly the word *tolerance*, tends to imply that other people are essentially a nuisance, and disguises the fact that we need and depend on each other. "They aren't blind," my son says of moles, "they just can't see." The same could be said of humans. We often manage not to see that we are, as Martin Luther King reminds us, "caught in an inescapable network of mutuality."

Even the Danger Model, which does not imagine discrimination as the most essential function of our immune system, can still be used to imagine a homicidal police force into our bodies. But scientists are already proposing that we may someday respond to infection by nurturing desirable bacteria rather than killing undesirables. We may fight disease without fighting. The article where I learned this is headlined "Tending the Body's Microbial Garden." Our bodies are not war machines that attack everything foreign and unfamiliar, this metaphor suggests, but gardens where, under the right conditions, we live in balance with many other organisms. In the garden of the body, we look inward and find not self, but other.

"We must cultivate our garden," Candide says in the last line of Voltaire's *Candide*, which is subtitled *or, Optimism*. The word *optimism* was new in 1759, and referred to the philosophy that this world, having been fashioned by God, is the best of all possible worlds. In *Candide*, Voltaire pokes fun at this variety of optimism, along with everything else. Not even reason and rationalism—those foundations of the Enlightenment thinking for which Voltaire is remembered—are spared. Rationalism, *Candide* suggests, can be irrational. And it is possible to employ reason while remaining decidedly unenlightened.

When the young Candide begins his romp around the world, it is easy for him to embrace optimism because he has lived a comfortable life. As he travels, he witnesses wars, natural disasters, rapes, and hangings. He meets a slave who has lost a hand and a leg. "It is the price we pay for the sugar you eat in Europe," the slave tells him. "If this is the best of all possible worlds," Candide begins to wonder, "what must the others be like?" But the book has a happy ending. Candide and his friends —who have been imprisoned and prostituted, who have suffered syphilis and the plague — work together on a small plot of land where they enjoy the fruits of their garden.

The conclusion of *Candide* is masterful, according to Flaubert, because it is "as stupid as life itself." My sister and I both remember where we were when we read *Candide* for the first time, but neither of us is sure what to make of the ending. Or at least my sister is not sure at midnight, which is when I ask her to interpret *Candide*. "You should just say you don't know what it means," she advises me sleepily. I do not know what it means. I want it to mean that the garden in which we work when we are no longer optimistic is not a retreat from the world, but a place where we cultivate the world.

If we extend the metaphor of the garden to our social body, we might imagine ourselves as a garden within a garden. The outer garden is no Eden, and no rose garden either. It is as strange and various as the inner garden of our bodies, where we host fungi and viruses and bacteria of both "good" and "bad" dispositions. This garden is unbounded and unkempt, bearing both fruit and thorns. Perhaps we should call it a wilderness. Or perhaps *community* is sufficient. However we choose to think of the social body, we are each other's environment. Immunity is a shared space—a garden we tend together.

Notes

13   In one of its broader senses, the word *inoculate* means "to join
       or unite." More narrowly, it means to introduce a germ to the
       body of a person. Inoculation can include vaccination as well
       as variolation, intentionally infecting a person with smallpox
       to induce immunity. I have also seen the word used in a
       medical journal to describe the practice of putting a baby's
       fallen pacifier in one's own mouth before returning it to the
       baby—thus introducing one's own germs to the child.

13   After my son's birth, I found myself in constant conversation
       with other mothers and the subject of our conversation
       was often motherhood itself. These mothers helped
       me understand how expansive the questions raised by
       mothering really are. In recognition of the debt my thinking
       owes to them, I have chosen, throughout this book, to use
       the word *mothers* in places where I could have used the word
       parents. I am writing to and from the women who complicated
       the subject of immunization for me. This does not mean that
       I believe immunization is exclusively of concern to women,
       but only that I want to address other mothers directly. In
       a culture that relishes pitting women against each other in
       "mommy wars," I feel compelled to leave some traces on
       the page of another kind of argument. This is a productive,
       necessary argument—an argument that does not reduce us,
       as the diminutive *mommy* implies, and that does not resemble
       war.

16   *the fact that US vaccines did not contain squalene, she said, had been
       disputed elsewhere:* In 1997, a series of stories in *Insight on the
       News* magazine suggested that Gulf War syndrome might
       be linked to the presence of squalene, among other things,
       in the anthrax vaccine. There was no squalene added to the
       anthrax vaccine, according to the FDA and the Department
       of Defense, but some laboratory tests were able to detect
       minuscule traces of the substance. In a test conducted by the
       FDA, researchers suspected that the source of these traces
       was the people doing the testing. "Because of the difficulty
       of removing squalene-containing fingerprint oils from
       laboratory glassware," they explained, "it is hard to know
       whether the squalene is truly present in some lots of the
       vaccine or is introduced by the testing process itself."

18   The metaphors I began hearing around vaccination when my
       son was an infant inspired me to reread Susan Sontag's essay

...   *Illness as Metaphor.* And then I read, for the first time, the essay she wrote a decade later, *AIDS and Its Metaphors.* "Of course, one cannot think without metaphors," she reminds us in this essay. Her project in *Illness as Metaphor,* she clarifies, was not to argue against metaphor, but to free cancer of burdensome metaphors that obscured, rather than revealed, truths about that disease.

"The people who get to impose their metaphors on the culture get to define what we consider to be true," George Lakoff and Mark Johnson write in *Metaphors We Live By.* My thinking about metaphor was informed by their book, and by *I Is an Other: The Secret Life of Metaphor and How It Shapes the Way We See the World* by James Geary. I reread *AIDS and Its Metaphors* many times over the years that I spent working on this book, and I consider Sontag one of the mothers with whom I conversed while I wrote.

18   Human papillomavirus is the most common sexually transmitted disease in the United States and the world, and it is the sole cause of cervical cancer. The CDC's 2006 recommendation that all girls should be vaccinated against HPV at age eleven or twelve led to widely reported concerns that the vaccine itself would encourage teenagers to become sexually active. A 2012 study published in *Pediatrics,* "Sexual Activity-Related Outcomes after Human Papillomavirus Vaccination of 11-to 12-Year-Olds," found that promiscuity was not one of the side effects of the vaccine.

22   *He then goes on to evoke Mark Twain: "I heard once of an American who so defined faith: 'that which enables us to believe things which we know to be untrue'":* Stoker is paraphrasing Twain's famous quote, "Faith is believing what you know ain't so."

25   The term *herd immunity* was first used in 1923, by researchers investigating bacterial infections in mice. The concept itself had been recognized much earlier, though its implications were not fully appreciated until widespread vaccination revealed that, for example, immunizing less than 90 percent of a population against diphtheria could reduce the incidence of disease by 99.99 percent. "That indirect protection occurs is obvious, both in logic and in observation," the epidemiologist Paul Fine notes in his review of the literature on herd immunity, "Herd Immunity: History, Theory, Practice." He goes on to explain that apparent exceptions to herd immunity do not refute the general principle, but only reveal that herd immunity can be fragile in

...   certain circumstances.

29   *A number of friends had offered his name when I asked for a recomm-*
endation, and so had my midwife, who referred to him as "left of
center": We had already abandoned my son's first pediatrician
for a new doctor by the time it occurred to me that the first
pediatrician had been recommended to me almost solely
because he did not ask his patients to follow the standard
immunization schedule. It was this that defined him as "left
of center," though his attitudes struck me as more typical of
right-wing politics.

31   Unless otherwise noted, all my disease statistics throughout
this book were drawn from the CDC or the WHO.

31   Before the vaccine for hep B was introduced, the disease
infected 200,000 people a year, and about a million
Americans were chronically infected. Rates of hep B
infection have declined by 82 percent since the routine
vaccination of newborns began in 1991, but somewhere
between 800,000 and 1.4 million people in the United States
are still chronically infected.

31   The risk of contracting hep B from a blood transfusion is
extremely minimal—the Red Cross estimates it at between 1
in 200,000 and 1 in 500,000. While very small, that risk is
probably greater than the risk of an infant having a serious
allergic reaction to the hep B vaccine—the CDC estimates
that risk as about 1 in 1.1 million.
   The possibility, however remote, that I could have
contracted hep B from a blood transfusion and passed it
to my newborn son was alarming when it first occurred to
me, but what ultimately disturbed me more was how many
factors I had failed to consider when I made the decision
not to vaccinate my son. I had not thought of his health in
relationship to my health, or the health of our community at
large.

31   *When the last nationwide smallpox epidemic began in 1898, some*
people believed that whites were not susceptible to the disease: A
new, milder strain of smallpox was circulating during this
epidemic, as Michael Willrich notes in *Pox: An American*
History, and it was sometimes confused with chicken pox or
taken for a new disease. As a new disease, it was associated
with outsiders and immigrants, hence the names "Cuban
itch," "Porto Rico scratch," "Manila scab," "Filipino itch,"

...   "Nigger itch," "Italian itch," and "Hungarian itch."

32   *Debates over vaccination, then as now, are often cast as debates over the integrity of science, though they could just as easily be understood as conversations about power:* In his history of smallpox at the turn of the century, Michael Willrich suggests that some of America's efforts toward colonization were made possible, in part, through vaccination. The vaccination campaigns in the Philippines and Puerto Rico were conducted ostensibly for the health of the natives, with this becoming eventually a justification for an ongoing colonial presence, but they also had the effect of making those places safe for colonizers. Vaccination by force was made illegal in the Philippines only after millions of people had been vaccinated by the US military.

32   *Britain's 1853 provision for free, mandatory vaccination:* This compulsory vaccination law, Nadja Durbach notes in her book *Bodily Matters: The Antivaccination Movement in England, 1853–1907*, was rarely enforced until 1867, when another vaccination act clarified the penalties for refusing to vaccinate.

33   "Stop Coddling the Super-rich," the *New York Times* headlined Warren Buffett's 2011 call for tax reform. Our tax system is just one of the many mechanisms by which we collectively protect the most privileged among us while we neglect the more vulnerable. "These and other blessings are showered upon us by legislators in Washington," Buffett wrote, "who feel compelled to protect us, much as if we were spotted owls or some other endangered species."

33   *Think of the unvaccinated boy in San Diego, for instance, who returned from a trip to Switzerland in 2008 with a case of measles that infected his two siblings, five schoolmates, and four children in his doctor's waiting room:* According to a 2010 study published in *Pediatrics*, "Measles Outbreak in a Highly Vaccinated Population, San Diego, 2008: Role of the Intentionally Undervaccinated," the public-sector cost of containing this outbreak was $124,517. That does not include the $14,458 in medical expenses for the infant who was hospitalized for three days, or the lost wages and other expenses of the families whose unvaccinated children were placed under a twenty-one-day quarantine after exposure. "Despite high community vaccination coverage," the study concluded, "measles outbreaks can occur among clusters of intentionally

... undervaccinated children, at major cost to public health agencies, medical systems, and families."

37 *Some of our white blood cells recombine their genetic material like random number generators, shuffling their sequences to create an immense variety of cells capable of recognizing an immense variety of pathogens:* No single person, I learned from the immunologist who explained this "recombinant" process to me, has the genetic material to respond to all diseases, but collectively humans have enough genetic diversity for humankind to survive any disease.

40 *A comprehensive report on vaccine "adverse events" was released in 2011 by a committee of eighteen medical experts who reviewed 12,000 studies of vaccination for the Institute of Medicine:* This report is titled "Adverse Effects of Vaccines: Evidence and Causality" and can be downloaded in full from the Institute of Medicine's website. The committee examined 158 possible adverse effects of vaccination, but found convincing evidence of only 9 adverse effects, 4 of which were related to contracting chicken pox from the chicken pox vaccine.

Over the two years it took to assess all the scientific evidence available to them, the committee worked without compensation. When I asked the chair of the committee, Ellen Clayton, what motivated them, she responded, "I was going to say the goodness of their hearts, and it's that too, but the other part is that it's an opportunity to contribute to policy making in the United States. There's a strong history of the policy makers around vaccination relying heavily on a series of reports from the Institute of Medicine."

The Institute of Medicine is an independent, nonprofit research organization whose mission is to help government officials and the public make healthcare decisions based on reliable information. Its members, medical professionals elected by their peers, donate their time and expertise to the institute's studies. Members who sit on committees are screened for conflicts of interest and their work is examined by outside experts. In 1986, Congress assigned the task of periodically reviewing the risks of vaccination to the Institute of Medicine. The 2011 report was the result of the twelfth such review, and the largest study to date.

41 The interplay between Paul Slovic and Cass Sunstein in "The Laws of Fear," Sunstein's review of Slovic's book *The Perception of Risk*, is compelling in part because the two are working from the same information, but drawing different

... conclusions. Slovic is more generous to the average person, and more interested in examining the complex value systems that make the risk assessments of lay people so unlike the risk assessments of experts. Sunstein is less patient, particularly in cases where faulty risk assessments by the general public may lead to increased risk.

Ordinary people, Sunstein observes, tend to make some ordinary errors when thinking about risk. We exaggerate the risk of unfamiliar things, and minimize the risk of familiar things. We also have a tendency, as Slovic found in his studies, to believe that risky things carry little benefit and that beneficial things carry little risk. Our sense that hand sanitizer poses us little risk may inflate how effective we believe it to be. And if we believe that vaccines carry a high risk, we may also tend to believe they are ineffective.

42 *Bicycles, the* New York Times *reports, "are involved in more accidents than any other consumer product, but beds rank a close second":* The information in this article by Sam Roberts, "Who Americans Are and What They Do, in Census Data," was drawn from the Census Bureau's 2007 Statistical Abstract of the United States. The raw data contained in the abstract's tables can be misleading, as Roberts notes: "The table of consumer products involved in injuries does not explain, for example, that one reason nearly as many injuries involve beds as bicycles is that more people use beds."

45 *One of the appeals of alternative medicine is that it offers not just an alternative philosophy or an alternative treatment but also an alternative language:* I do not intend to suggest that there are not other reasons why we turn to alternative medicine, but I am interested in how the marketing of alternative medicine exploits our fears. This marketing is not without its ironies, as when the chemicals used to cleanse the body of toxins in chelation therapy prove to be toxic.

Alternative medicine in this country has its roots in the Popular Health Movement of the 1830s. This movement was, as Barbara Ehrenreich and Deirdre English write in *For Her Own Good*, a response to both the professionalization of medicine and the dangers of early nineteenth-century medicine. A number of alternative practices emerged during this period, including homeopathy and hydropathy, as well as Sylvester Graham's system of eating whole grains and fresh vegetables and avoiding all drugs and herbal remedies. With the exception of homeopaths, who often embraced vaccination because it supported their theory that "like cures

...   like," many alternative health practitioners were expressly
      opposed to vaccination.

      The most popular alternative practice was promoted
      by Samuel Thomson, who wanted to free medicine from
      the marketplace and democratize it so that each person
      could be his or her own healer. Nearly a quarter of all
      Americans subscribed to this philosophy at its height, but
      by the end of the 1830s Thomsonians had, as Ehrenreich
      and English write, "succumbed to the very forces they had
      set out to challenge. Where once they had denouncedthe
      transformation of healing into a commodity, now they sought
      to package their own alternative into a new commodity."

      This legacy lives on in our contemporary alternative
      health movement, which promotes vitamins and supplements
      that cost Americans $30 billion a year, are produced by some
      of the same companies that produce pharmaceuticals, and
      amount to a large—and largely unregulated—industry.

45   Commentators on national television were insisting that
      same-sex marriage was "unnatural" even on the day
      the Supreme Court determined that a key provision of
      the Defense of Marriage Act was unconstitutional. This
      decision, Justice Antonin Scalia argued in his dissent, sprang
      from a "diseased root." Clearly, there is a punitive moralism
      hiding behind both our understanding of what is natural and
      what it means to be diseased.

46   *"In the pharmaceutical world," the writer Jane Smith observes, "the
      great division is between biologicals and chemicals":* In her book
      Patenting the Sun: Polio and the Salk Vaccine, Smith expands on
      this further: "Biologicals are tricky to produce, expensive to
      store, and easy to get wrong." Drug companies, she notes, get
      out of the business of biologicals whenever they can. "They
      live off the chemicals. Chemicals let you sleep easy at night
      and wake up rich in the morning."

48   *Carson may have overstated some of the dangers of DDT:* In *The
      Green Crusade: Rethinking the Roots of Environmentalism*, the
      political scientist Charles Rubin details a few cases in which
      Rachel Carson distorted her information or misrepresented
      her sources. She cited a letter to the editor of a medical
      journal, for example, as if it were a scientific report. And
      she implied that a study on leukemia had led to conclusions
      that were counter to the conclusions the author of the study
      had made. Carson did not misrepresent all her sources, as
      Rubin makes clear, but her case was not as unequivocal as

...   she made it seem.

52   *I understood it as a broader question of belonging:* As a poet who writes in prose, or a prose writer informed by poetry, I have often found myself confronted with the question of belonging.The problem has not been finding a place where I belong, which is how a children's book might tell it, but of finding ways of insisting on belonging nowhere. To this end, I have tried to heed Alice Walker's lines "Be nobody's darling; / Be an outcast." The tradition of the personal essay is full of self-appointed outcasts. In that tradition, I am not a poet or the press, but an essayist, a citizen thinker.

55   *And perhaps we have never been modern, either:* The anthropologist Bruno Latour's book *We Have Never Been Modern* is what Haraway is referencing when she writes, "We have never been human."

60   "The body is not a battlefield," Susan Sontag warns in *AIDS and Its Metaphors.* Bad metaphors, she contends, can disrupt our understanding of our bodies. Not all metaphors distort illness equally, and not all are damaging, but Sontag finds the war metaphor uniquely destructive. "It overmobilizes, it overdescribes, and it powerfully contributes to the excommunicating and stigmatizing of the ill," she writes. "Give it back to the war-makers."

67   *a report on vaccine side effects, which concluded its brief historical overview of child mortality with the observation that now "children are expected to survive to adulthood":* This is from "Adverse Effects of Vaccines: Evidence and Causality" (see note to page 40), which notes that in 1900, in the United States, 100 out of every 1,000 babies would die before their first birthdays, and 5 more would die before the age of five. By 2007, those numbers had fallen to less than 7 out of every 1,000 babies who would die before their first birthdays, and only .29 more before the age of five. "Diseases severe enough to kill children and adults can also leave survivors disabled in some way," the report observes, "and as mortality has fallen, so has the chance of severe disability from these diseases."

73   Most of my information and much of my thinking about the history of women and medicine was drawn from *For Her Own Good: Two Centuries of the Experts' Advice to Women* by Barbara Ehrenreich and Deirdre English. I also relied on their earlier

...   book *Witches, Midwives, and Nurses: A History of Women Healers.*
The introduction to the second edition of that book quotes
the historian John Demos, who observes that a quarter
to a third of the women tried for witchcraft in colonial
New England were known for their abilities as healers or
midwives. "The underlying linkage here is obvious enough,"
Demos writes. "The ability to heal and the ability to harm
seemed intimately related." As, I would argue, they still do.

75   *an investigative journalist discovered that Wakefield had been
paid for his research by a lawyer preparing a lawsuit against a
vaccine manufacturer:* This journalist was Brian Deer, and
the amount Wakefield was paid by Richard Barr's law firm
was $800,000. In pursuit of evidence for a lawsuit, this
firm gave $10 million to doctors and scientists researching
a link between vaccination and autism. In *Autism's False
Prophets,* Paul Offit details where that money went. Over $1
million went to Unigenetics Limited, the company that tested
Wakefield's samples. Kenneth Aitken, a pathologist who
argued for Britain to change its vaccination policy based
on Wakefield's research, received $400,000. And Marcel
Kinsbourne, a neurologist who supported Wakefield's
hypothesis, received $800,000.

80   Barbara Loe Fisher is president of the National Vaccine
Information Center, which is not, as its name might suggest,
a federal agency. "Its relationship with the US government,"
the journalist Michael Specter writes, "consists almost
entirely of opposing federal efforts aimed at vaccinating
children." In the spring of 2011, a CBS jumbotron in Times
Square began displaying an advertisement with the image
of a woman cradling an infant next to the words *Vaccines:
Know the risks.* This was followed by the word *Vaccination*
superimposed over the Statue of Liberty along with the
tagline "Your Health. Your family. Your choice." The logo
and website address for the NVIC, present on the screen for
the entire ad, then filled the frame.

The educational materials compiled on the NVIC website
suggest that vaccination may cause, among other things,
autism and diabetes. "Taking what NVIC says about
vaccines at face value," the physician and journalist Rahul
Parikh observes, "is akin to believing Joe Camel when he
tells you that smoking doesn't cause lung cancer." This might
seem at first like a flawed comparison, in that antivaccine
activists do not appear to be selling a product. But fear is
an intangible that sells any number of products, and the

...   possibility that someone has a vested interest in widespread
fear of vaccination is evidenced in the Times Square ad itself,
which includes on every frame the website address for the
cosponsor, the physician Joseph Mercola.

Mercola runs the Mercola Natural Health Center in
the suburbs of Chicago, though he himself no longer sees
patients. Since 2006, he has devoted most of his time to
his website, which hosts articles on the dangers of water
fluoridation, metal amalgam dental fillings, and vaccines,
with numerous forays into less-traveled terrain including
a theory that AIDS is not caused by HIV. This site draws
about 1.9 million visitors per month, as Bryan Smith
observes in his article "Dr. Mercola: Visionary or Quack?"
The products available for purchase range from tanning beds
to air purifiers to vitamins and supplements. The website
and Mercola LLC generated an estimated $7 million in
2010, and in 2011 Mercola donated $1 million to a number of
organizations, including the NVIC.

81   Jenny McCarthy, who maintains that she is not antivaccine
but "anti-toxins" led a 2008 march in Washington, DC,
organized around the theme "Green Our Vaccines." The
march and its slogan, which the physician David Gorski calls
"wonderfully Orwellian," illustrate how modes of resistance
can be coopted for purposes other than meaningful
resistance. McCarthy's antivaccine movement borrows
from the rhetoric of environmentalism without engaging in
environmentalist action, in the same manner that the earlier
antivaccine movement in Britain borrowed from the rhetoric
of abolitionism without engaging in abolitionist action.

84   For quite some time, all I knew about the complication I
suffered following my son's birth was that it is called uterine
inversion and that it is very rare. It is also, apparently,
featured on the final episode of the television show *ER*, which
my midwife discouraged me from watching because the
woman with uterine inversion dies in surgery after giving
birth. When I asked the obstetrician who operated on me
whether I should expect this complication to happen again
with another baby, she told me that nobody knows enough
to say for sure. My midwife, who had attended thousands of
births, had never witnessed a uterine inversion before my
son's birth. Several years would pass before I would learn
that this particular complication happens in about 1 out of
3,000 births. And in around 15 percent of those cases, the
mother dies.

88 *Privilege, too, is a positional good, and some have argued that health is as well:* The concept of positional goods was explained to me by my sister, who referred me to an article by Harry Brighouse and Adam Swift titled "Equality, Priority, and Positional Goods." This article explains that health, unlike education, is not widely understood as a positional good. "In fact, however, one's health does have competitive value," the authors argue. "Fit and healthy people are, other things being equal, more likely to succeed in the competition for jobs and other scarce goods. Indeed, some social scientists have suggested that health is an important element in the complicated causal story that explains why economically successful parents tend to have economically successful children. Children of wealthy parents tend to be healthier than children of poor parents, and their being so helps to explain why they do better at school and in the labor market. If that is so, and health is indeed a determinant of children's differential chances of achieving better or worse rewarded occupational positions, then health does indeed have a competitive, and hence positional, aspect. The value to me of my health does depend on how healthy others are. In the land of the blind, the one-eyed man is king."

89 *Thirty years after routine vaccination for smallpox ceased in the United States, the government asked researchers at the University of Iowa to test the remaining stores of the vaccine for efficacy:* President George W. Bush was vaccinated against smallpox in 2002, as part of a plan to immunize 10 million police and health workers. This plan was never realized, in part because of resistance from public health officials, nurses' unions, and hospitals. "The president's vaccination was a highly politicized public health gesture, a symbolic act demonstrating that Saddam Hussein's capabilities and plans were real and evil enough to justify aggression against his regime," Arthur Allen writes in his book *Vaccine: The Controversial Story of Medicine's Greatest Lifesaver.* The government had no evidence that Saddam had access to smallpox, but the possibility that he might was used to justify both a dubious vaccination campaign and the invasion of Iraq. "This was how we came," Allen writes, "at the beginning of the twenty-first century, to vaccinate our president against an extinct disease."

102 *Vaccination allows us to use the products of capitalism for purposes that are counter to the pressures of capital:* In the last line of

...   "Paranoid Reading and Reparative Reading, or, You're So
Paranoid, You Probably Think This Essay Is About You,"
from her book *Touching Feeling: Affect, Pedagogy, Performativity*,
Eve Sedgwick points hopefully toward what we can learn
from "the many ways selves and communities succeed in
extracting sustenance from the objects of a culture—even of
a culture whose avowed desire has often been not to sustain
them."

104   If *paternalism* is a dirty word, *maternalism* is also somewhat
soiled by its association with a time period in which women
had to justify their work as activists by arguing that they
were "naturally" inclined to protect other people. "By the
latter 19th century in the United States, maternalism began
to take on sociopolitical connotations," Carolyn Weber
writes in her entry on *maternalism* for the *Encyclopedia of
Gender and Society*, "so that the term came to denote a school
of activism in which women, to fight for public causes,
appealed to the qualities they believed were inherent to their
gender. As a result, maternalists are seen as women who take
mothering outside the home and into their communities for
the larger social good."

111   *the ways in which having access to one's own cord blood might be
advantageous later in life are still fairly limited:* Most children
who receive cord blood transplants need blood from a donor,
rather than their own cord blood, which may carry the
very condition they are being treated for. This is one of the
advantages of public cord blood banking noted by Ruben
Rucoba, a pediatrician whose own infant daughter received a
lifesaving transplant from a public bank. In his 2010 article
"Public Cord Banks Offer Many Advantages over Private
Banks," Rucoba observes that public banks participate in
a national registry, so blood donated to these banks will
very likely be used by someone who needs it. Blood stored
in private banks is likely to go unused, as the chance that a
child will need her own cord blood is somewhere around 1
in 200,000. And while public banks are required to meet
stringent federal standards, private banks are not. The
American Academy of Pediatrics issued a statement against
private cord blood banking in 2007, expressing concerns
that private banks were taking advantage of parents by
selling them an unproven, unnecessary service.

112   A 2011 survey published in *Pediatrics*, "Alternative

... Vaccination Schedule Preferences among Parents of Young Children," found that more than one in ten parents were using an alternative vaccination schedule. And of the parents who were following the schedule recommended by the CDC, over a quarter thought that delaying vaccination would be safer. These parents, the researchers concluded, were "at risk" for switching to an alternative schedule.

112 *there is no credible evidence, beyond Dr. Bob's personal speculations, that spacing and delaying vaccinations minimizes the incidence of side effects:* After an investigation designed to address the concerns of parents, advocacy groups, and the media, among others, about the childhood immunization schedule, the Institute of Medicine released a 2013 report titled "The Childhood Immunization Schedule and Safety: Stakeholder Concerns, Scientific Evidence, and Future Studies." This report found no compelling rationale for following alternative schedules, and concluded, "The committee found no significant evidence to imply that the recommended immunization schedule is not safe. Furthermore, existing surveillance and response systems have identified known adverse events associated with vaccination. The federal research infrastructure is a strong system."

113 *Tetanus is not a disease that affects infants, according to Dr. Bob:* The spores of tetanus bacteria live in the soil everywhere, and anyone, including infants, can contract tetanus from dirt introduced into a wound. In developing countries, many newborns contract tetanus through their unhealed umbilical cords. Deaths from tetanus in this country have declined over 99 percent since shortly after the vaccine became available in 1938, and neonatal tetanus has been nearly eliminated. This is owed in part to improved childbirth practices, and also to the maternal antibodies that temporarily protect babies born to women who have been vaccinated. Between 2001 and 2008, only one newborn contracted tetanus in the United States.

113 *Hib disease is rare:* Many people harbor the Hib bacteria in their noses and throats, but are immune to it. Before the introduction of the Hib vaccine in 1985, infection with *Haemophilus influenzae* type b was the most common cause of meningitis in this country. About 1 in every 200 children under five years old developed invasive Hib disease, and over 15,000 children suffered Hib meningitis every year.

113   *measles is not that bad:* In this country, one out of every twenty children who contract measles will develop pneumonia, the complication that most often leads to death. The case fatality rate for measles fluctuates depending on a number of factors including age—the disease is most fatal in children under five and adults. Between the years 1987 and 1992, about 3 in every 1,000 cases of measles in the United States resulted in death, but the case fatality rate for this country is usually estimated at about 1 in 1,000.

116   *Infants are exposed to an onslaught of bacteria the moment they leave the womb, even before they exit the birth canal:* There are between 2,000 and 6,000 immunological components—the proteins that evoke an immune response—in a single bacterium. The smallpox vaccine, in comparison, contains about 200 immunological components.

117   *a website that also compiles evidence that the Holocaust was a hoax and that anti-Semitism was invented by Zionists:* This website is whale.to, which enjoys a high ranking in Google searches for "vaccination." It hosts, among many other curiosities, the full text of the *Protocols of the Elders of Zion*, a document pretending to be the minutes of a meeting among Jewish leaders planning to take over the world through control of the economy and the press.

117   *Handley, a venture capitalist, is the cofounder of a private equity firm with over $1 billion under management as well as the cofounder of Generation Rescue, an autism advocacy organization:* Shortly after its inception in 2005, Generation Rescue publicized the theory that vaccines cause autism through a media campaign that included full-page ads in the *New York Times* and *USA Today*. Jenny McCarthy served as their spokeswoman and is now their president.

117   *Some parents of autistic children consider this exploitation:* A number of these parents—including Kathleen Seidel, who founded the website neurodiversity.com, and Camille Clark, otherwise known as Autism Diva—are profiled by Paul Offit in *Autism's False Prophets*.

122   What exactly constituted the real thing, when it came to medicine, was a question of considerable complexity in the early nineteenth century. Medicine at that time was practiced by bonesetters, midwives, herbalists, and a range of other lay healers in addition to "regular" doctors, who were

... themselves a motley crew. There was no central licensing body for doctors, no set standards for practice, and medical degrees could be openly purchased.

As doctors struggled to establish medicine as a legitimate profession and to regulate its practice, Nadja Durbach writes in *Bodily Matters*, they appealed to the state for exclusive authority over vaccination. An association of British doctors issued a report in 1840 complaining that vaccination was being provided by "itinerating quacks, petty tradesmen of an inferior order, blacksmiths, excisemen, druggists, &c; the poor, one with another." Vaccination was being provided, in other words, by everyone who provided medical care.

The right to perform vaccination was eventually restricted to physicians and state-licensed vaccinators, and variolation was made illegal in Britain in 1841. While this allowed for better regulation of immunization, it also reinforced fears that the state was colluding with doctors to create a profit-driven monopoly over medicine. With this legislation, Durbach observes, resistance to the professionalization and standardization of medicine also became resistance to government authority.

124 *The clause was rather vague, requiring only that the objector "satisfy" a magistrate that her objection was a matter of conscience:* There was some debate at the time over whether women could or should apply for conscientious exemption, as men were the legal guardians of their children and it was not appropriate for women, according to one politician, to exercise their conscience outside the home. The law itself used the word *parent* and did not exclude women, but in some places women were turned away and told that only fathers could apply. In other places, almost all applicants were women. Eventually, an ambiguous amendment was interpreted to include women. "As a result of this interpretation of the new legislation," Nadja Durbach writes, "the first widely acknowledged conscientious objectors were not only predominantly working class but also often female."

126 *We have them to thank for the fact that we can no longer be vaccinated at gunpoint:* We also owe some of the safety of our current vaccine schedule to the parents who refused vaccination during a smallpox epidemic in 1901 (more on this in the note to page 137); to the parents who appealed to Congress for better tracking of vaccine side effects in 1984 (that group of parents would become the NVIC—see the note to page 80); and to parents like John Salamone,

... who successfully advocated for the oral polio vaccine to
be replaced with a safer inactivated polio vaccine in 1998.
Advocacy for vaccine safety is not the same as antivaccine
activism that aims to undermine, rather than improve, our
system of vaccination. But some groups, like the NVIC,
engage in both.

127 *And allowing oneself to remain vulnerable to disease remains a legal
privilege today:* The word *privilege* is from the Latin *privilegium*,
meaning "law applying to one person." A legal exemption
from vaccination is, by definition, a privilege. Vaccination
is required for admission to public schools as well as many
day care facilities and pre-schools in the United States.
Every state in the country offers medical exemptions to this
requirement, all but two states offer religious exemptions,
and nineteen states offer philosophical exemptions, our
version of the conscientious objection.

128 *But the exact number of people this might be—the threshold at which
herd immunity is lost and the risk of disease rises dramatically for
both the vaccinated and the unvaccinated—varies depending on the
disease and the vaccine and the population in question:* In "'Herd
Immunity': A Rough Guide," Paul Fine argues that we must
be "wary of target thresholds for vaccination, insofar as
thresholds are based on assumptions that greatly simplify the
complexity of actual populations. In most circumstances, the
sensible public health practice is to aim for 100% coverage,
with all the doses recommended, recognizing that 100% is
never achievable, hoping to reach whatever is the 'real' herd
immunity threshold in the population concerned."

136 *As the Environmental Protection Agency observed at the time,
Corexit was neither the safest nor the most effective dispersant on
the market—it was simply the most readily available to BP in the
wake of the spill:* Before the spill, the EPA rated Corexit as less
effective and more toxic than at least twelve other products.
But after the spill, theEPA conducted a test that found that
Corexit mixed with Louisiana crude was no more or less
toxic to marine life than other dispersants mixed with oil.
One of the EPA's own employees questioned the merit of
this test, as Suzanne Goldenberg noted in an article for the
Guardian, "BP Oil Spill: Obama Administration's Scientists
Admit Alarm over Chemicals." And Susan Shaw, the
director of the Marine Environmental Research Institute,
told the *Guardian*, "It was only one test and it was very crude."
By that point, the amount of Corexit that had been used in

...   the Gulf already constituted, as the toxicologist Ron Kendall observed, an enormous unregulated "eco-toxicological experiment." The results of that experiment are still to be concluded.

137   *"In the fall of 1901, regulation was a controversial idea," the historian Michael Willrich writes. "A few months later, it was federal law." What happened in between was a smallpox outbreak in Camden, New Jersey:* When smallpox broke out in Camden, the Board of Education announced that children who were not vaccinated could not attend school. Thousands of schoolchildren were vaccinated over the next month, but then a sixteen-year-old boy who had recently been vaccinated came down with a case of tetanus that locked his jaw and sent his body into convulsions. And then a sixteen-year-old girl who had recently been vaccinated came down with tetanus, and an eleven-year-old boy who had recently been vaccinated died less than a day after coming down with tetanus.

Nearly all the afflicted children, an investigation would find, had received vaccines from the same manufacturer. And this manufacturer would also be linked to an outbreak of tetanus at Philadelphia Hospital. In Europe, vaccines were controlled or even produced by governments, but here anyone could make and sell a vaccine. The smallpox vaccine was sourced from cows and produced on farms, where it was prone to contamination from the dust and manure of the stables, which often contained tetanus bacilli.

As deaths from tetanus began to exceed deaths from smallpox in Camden, parents launched a school strike and refused vaccination. When isolated cases of tetanus were reported in schoolchildren who had been vaccinated in Atlantic City and Philadelphia, the Camden panic became a national crisis. With resistance to vaccination rising, Theodore Roosevelt signed the Biologics Control Act, which established a system of licensing and inspection for vaccine manufacturers. This legislation, the *New York Times* observed, "would involve a dangerous expansion of Federal authority were it not aimed to correct an evil yet more dangerous."

The danger, as many understood it, was not just that children might be harmed by bad vaccines, but that even more children might be harmed by smallpox when their parents justifiably refused vaccination. In Camden, a total of nine children died of tetanus after vaccination, and fifteen people—none of them recently vaccinated—died of smallpox. "By the time the epidemic wound down that spring," Willrich writes, "smallpox had indeed proved more fatal

...   there than vaccination."

138   *Vaccines are subject to ongoing surveillance through a national database:* The Vaccine Adverse Event Reporting System (VAERS) collects reports of "adverse events" (including everything from fevers and rashes to seizures and anaphylaxis) following vaccination. This system is sometimes misunderstood as a database of vaccine side effects, but it is intended to function as a passive surveillance system in which clusters or patterns of similar reports will prompt further investigation by the CDC. Anyone can make a report to VAERS, including parents and personal injury lawyers, and the database inevitably gathers reports of events unrelated to vaccination—deaths from suicides and car accidents following vaccination have been reported to VAERS, as well as one man's transformation into the Incredible Hulk following his vaccination against influenza.

   In July of 1999, CDC officials became alarmed by fifteen VAERS reports of babies who had developed an uncommon form of intestinal blockage called intussusception after receiving a new rotavirus vaccine, RotaShield. (This was not the rotavirus vaccine coinvented by Paul Offit.) The CDC had recommended the vaccine for all infants because rotavirus was responsible for 70,000 hospitalizations and sixty deaths in this country every year. When VAERS raised suspicion of a potential problem, the CDC suspended use of the vaccine and launched an investigation. The RotaShield vaccine had been available for less than a year at that point. By October, researchers had concluded that children who received the vaccine were twenty-five times more likely to develop intussusception than those who did not, and the vaccine was taken off the market. The risk of developing intussusception after vaccination had been about 1 in 10,000 and VAERS had served to detect that risk within months.

142   *Robbed of their context, some of the components involved in vaccine production—human albumin, protein fragments from human cells, residual DNA—suggest that debris from other bodies is being injected into us:* I drew these particular examples from the many lists of vaccine components in *The Vaccine Book* by Robert Sears.

143   *"Is the immune system at the heart of a new incarnation of social Darwinism that allows people of different 'quality' to be distinguished from each other?" asks the anthropologist Emily Martin:* Martin does not ask this question in the context of vaccination

   ...   specifically, but in a wider context of American attitudes toward health and disease in general. This question, which opens the final chapter of her book *Flexible Bodies: Tracking Immunity in American Culture—From the Days of Polio to the Age of AIDS*, is informed by her observations around AIDS and emergent diseases, as well as late capitalism and racism. "It is clear to me," she writes, "that what is at stake in our understanding of 'health' are the broadest issues of the survival and death of the social order itself."

144   *Siddhartha Mukherjee's history of cancer, in which he argues not only that life causes cancer but that cancer is us*: In *The Emperor of All Maladies: A Biography of Cancer*, Mukherjee suggests, "We tend to think of cancer as a 'modern' illness because its metaphors are so modern." Cancer, he explains, "is an age-related disease—sometimes exponentially so. The risk of breast cancer, for instance, is about 1 in 400 for a thirty-year-old woman and increases to 1 in 9 for a seventy-year-old." And, "Nineteenth-century doctors often linked cancer to civilization: cancer, they imagined, was caused by the rush and whirl of modern life, which somehow incited pathological growth in the body. The link was correct, but the causality was not: civilization did not cause cancer, but by extending human life spans—civilization unveiled it."

145   The "Vaccine Court" was established by the National Childhood Vaccine Injury Act in 1986, the same legislation that provided for the independent review of vaccine safety by the Institute of Medicine and created a system for reporting vaccine side effects through VAERS.

    The chain of events that led to this legislation began in 1981, when a British study suggested that the whole-cell pertussis component of the DTP vaccine (diphtheria, tetanus, and whole-cell pertussis), which has now been replaced by an acellular pertussis component, could cause permanent brain damage. As Paul Offit explains in his book *Deadly Choices*, this finding would be refuted by a number of later studies—an investigation by neuropathologists in England, an epidemiological study in Denmark, and a study of over 200,000 children in the United States—but not before fear of the DTP vaccine spread to the United States. In 1984 a television documentary, *DPT: Vaccine Roulette*, dramatized this fear with footage of severely disabled children and interviews with experts who warned that "the dangers are far greater than any doctors have been willing to admit." Its national broadcast was followed by a dramatic increase in

...   lawsuits against pharmaceutical companies.

"By 1985," Arthur Allen writes, "219 pertussis vaccine lawsuits had been filed in U.S. courts, with an average compensation re-quest of $26 million. When the lawsuits began in 1981, the total size of the pertussis vaccine market in the United States was only about $2 million." One of the three companies making DTP quit distribution and another stopped production because of liability. In 1986, the last company still making the vaccine announced that it would no longer continue production.

At a Senate hearing in 1984, a group of parents who would eventually call their organization the National Vaccine Information Center (see note to page 80) had asked the government to expand research on vaccine side effects, to require physicians to report side effects to a central database, and to create a compensation program for children who had been seriously injured by vaccines. Hoping to address not just the vaccine shortage, but also the concerns that had led to the litigation that contributed to it, legislators passed a bill that met these parents' requests. This bill was designed to protect the interests of both vaccine manufacturers and parents—predictably, neither liked it.

The National Childhood Vaccine Injury Act provided for the federal government, not vaccine makers, to be sued in cases of vaccine injury. Parents did not like this because they worried that manufacturers would not be held liable for the safety of their products. The act also provided for the parents of injured children to be compensated without definitively proving that the injury had been caused by a vaccine. Manufacturers did not like this because they were concerned that their products would become associated with side effects those products did not actually cause.

148   *as the medical researcher John Ioannidis has observed, "most published research findings are false":* Described in the *Boston Globe* as an "instant cult classic," Ioannidis's 2005 paper "Why Most Published Research Findings Are False" has been downloaded more times than any other technical paper published by the journal *PLOS Medicine*. Both of the scientists who read a draft of this book for me expressed concern that my quote of Ioannidis's bold title could be misleading. In many cases, as one of the scientists pointed out, the data in published research is correct, even when the conclusions drawn from that data are not. "Most published research needs refinement," would be more accurate than "most published research findings are false," he suggested.

...   In his 2007 study "Most Published Research Findings Are False—But a Little Replication Goes a Long Way," the CDC researcher Ramal Moonesinghe and his colleagues find that the likelihood of a research finding being true increases significantly after it has been replicated in several other studies. Or, as Carl Sagan puts it, "Science thrives on errors, cutting them away one by one."

151   *"A scientist is never certain," the scientist Richard Feynman reminds us:* Having contributed to the invention of the atomic bomb, Feynman had considerable occasion for uncertainty.

151   Keats: "'Beauty is truth, truth beauty,'—that is all / ye know on earth, and all ye need to know."

152   *Children with egg allergies can react to this particular vaccine, which is grown in eggs:* I have since learned that many children with egg allergies can safely receive the flu vaccine. My son was ultimately vaccinated despite his allergy.

157   The seasonal flu vaccine is unlike other vaccines in a number of ways, the most obvious being that it tends to be less effective. This is because influenza viruses change rapidly and different strains of influenza cause the flu each year. In order to prepare a vaccine in advance of flu season, researchers must make an educated guess about which strains of the virus are going to be active in the coming year. The match is usually good. But vaccinated people can be infected with other strains of influenza not covered by the vaccine. This leads some people to conclude that the vaccine does not work. It does work. Even in years when the vaccine is not a good match for the strains of the virus that are actually in circulation, it can still reduce the severity of the disease in vaccinated people and reduce the incidence of disease across the population as a whole. And people who have been vaccinated against the flu many times can carry a cumulative immunity to many strains of the flu.

     Both the efficacy of the flu vaccine and the severity of the flu virus fluctuate from year to year, making individual risk assessments difficult. The virus may be weak for many years in a row, producing mostly mild cases of influenza, and then a much more dangerous strain may suddenly emerge.

159   I introduced my son to the rules of baseball one spring day when we were playing on the beach with a Wiffle ball and a plastic bat. After his first "out" he began to understand that

··· we were not on the same team. "You're the bad guy," he said with a sly smile. He had recently discovered superheroes and the easy opposition between bad and good. He gravitated toward this opposition, but he was also drawn to the word *renegade*, which I defined for him as someone who breaks the rules for reasons that person believes are good. "Sometimes I'm a renegade," he confessed to me.

"I'm not a bad guy or a good guy," I told him. "I'm just on the other team." He laughed at this weak reasoning. I threw a pitch and he struck out. "Nice try, bad guy," he said to me amicably as he handed over the bat. He may not have fully understood the game, but he understood that I wanted him to hit the ball as much as he wanted to hit it. We were not really on different teams—we were playing together.

160 The poem "Poetry" by Marianne Moore begins, "I, too, dislike it: there are things that are important beyond/ all this fiddle. / Reading it, however, with a perfect contempt for it, one / discovers in / it after all, a place for the genuine."

Selected sources

Author's note: Hundreds of newspaper articles, countless scholarly articles, dozens of books, many blog posts, some poems, several novels, one immunology textbook, a handful of transcripts, piles of magazine clippings, and many essays fed my investigation of immunity. A full list of all the sources I consulted would be un-wieldy, but I would like to acknowledge those that were essential to my work. Listed below are the texts from which I have quoted without full attribution and the texts to which I am most indebted for information or ideas.

14   *That fall, the* New Yorker *ran an article ... it did not acknowledge any good reason for doubt:* "The Fear Factor," Michael Specter, *New Yorker,* October 12, 2009.

18   *The ability to make and understand basic metaphors ... "our metaphors prime how we think and act":* James Geary, *I Is an Other: The Secret Life of Metaphor and How It Shapes the Way We See the World* (New York: Harper, 2011), 155, 19, 100.

19   *"inappropriate for girls of such a young age":* Brian Brady, "Parents Block Plans to Vaccinate Nine-Year-Olds against Sex Virus," *Scotland on Sunday,* January 7, 2007.

19–20   *Throughout the nineteenth century ... bacterial contamination remained a problem:* Nadja Durbach, *Bodily Matters: The Anti--Vaccine Movement in England, 1853–1907* (Durham, NC: Duke University Press, 2005), 132, 118, 138–39.

25–27   *herd immunity:* Paul Fine, "Herd Immunity: History, Theory, Practice," *Epidemiologic Reviews,* July 1993; Paul Fine, "'Herd Immunity': A Rough Guide," *Clinical Infectious Diseases,* April 2011.

30   *In an article for* Mothering *magazine ... "she had no chance of catching":* Jennifer Margulis, "The Vaccine Debate," *Mothering,* July 2009.

30–31   *hep B:* Paul Offit, *Deadly Choices* (New York: Basic Books, 2011), 64–67; Stanley Plotkin et al., *Vaccines,* 6th ed. (New York: Elsevier, 2012), 205–34; Gregory Armstrong et al., "Childhood Hepatitis B Virus Infections in the United States before Hepatitis B Immunization," *Pediatrics,*

...   November 2001.

31–32   *When the last nationwide smallpox epidemic ... poor were enlisted in the protection of the privileged:* Michael Willrich, *Pox: An American History* (New York: Penguin, 2011), 41, 5, 58.

32–33   *Debates over vaccination ... it fell to the poor to articulate their vulnerability:* Nadja Durbach, *Bodily Matters: The Anti-Vaccine Movement in England, 1853–1907* (Durham, NC: Duke University Press, 2005), 83.

33   *a 2004 analysis of CDC data:* P. J. Smith et al., "Children Who Have Received No Vaccines: Who Are They and Where Do They Live?" *Pediatrics,* July 2004.

35   *We need germs ... one particular childhood disease that might prevent allergies:* David Strachan, "Family Size, Infection, and Atopy: The First Decade of the Hygiene Hypothesis," *Thorax,* August 2000.

36   *the overall diversity of germs in our environment ... the bacteria that colonize our skin, lungs, nose, throat, and gut:* Graham Rook, "A Darwinian View of the Hygiene or 'Old Friends' Hypothesis," *Microbe,* April 2012.

36–37   *a million different viruses in a teaspoon of seawater ... "There is no us and them":* Carl Zimmer, *A Planet of Viruses* (Chicago: University of Chicago Press, 2011), 47–52.

38–39   *triclosan:* Alliance for the Prudent Use of Antibiotics, "Triclosan," January 2011; Jia-Long Fang et al., "Occurrence, Efficacy, Metabolism, and Toxicity of Triclosan," *Journal of Environmental Science and Health,* September 20, 2010.

40–41   *Natural infections of measles, mumps, chicken pox, and influenza ... "favors rejection" of the theory that the MMR vaccine causes autism:* Ellen Clayton et al., "Adverse Effects of Vaccines: Evidence and Causality," Institute of Medicine, August 25, 2011.

42   *risk perception:* Cass Sunstein, "The Laws of Fear," *Harvard Law Review,* February 2002; Paul Slovic, "Perception of Risk," *Science,* April 1987.

43   *Paranoia, the theorist ... "some things well and others poorly":* Eve

...   Sedgwick, "Paranoid Reading and Reparative Reading, or, You're So Paranoid, You Probably Think This Essay Is About You," in *Touching Feeling: Affect, Pedagogy, Performativity* (Durham, NC: Duke University Press, 2003), 130–31.

43–44   *Intuitive toxicology ... less harmful than man-made chemicals:* Paul Slovic, *The Perception of Risk* (London: Earthscan Publications, 2000), 310–11.

45–46   *"Obviously ... There can be continuity between them, and there must be":* Wendell Berry, "Getting Along with Nature," in *Home Economics* (New York: North Point Press, 1987), 17, 25–26.

46   *"In the pharmaceutical world ... from chemical compounds":* Jane S. Smith, *Patenting the Sun: Polio and the Salk Vaccine* (New York: Morrow, 1990), 221.

46   *"Probably we're diseased ... hardly ever ill":* Emily Martin, *Flexible Bodies: Tracking Immunity in American Culture— from the Days of Polio to the Age of AIDS* (Boston: Beacon, 1994), 107.

48–49   *DDT is not exactly what Carson feared it was ... she got some things wrong:* Robert Zubrin, "The Truth about DDT and Silent Spring," *New Atlantis*, September 27, 2012.

49   *"Few books" ... "its eradication in rich ones":* Tina Rosenberg, "What the World Needs Now Is DDT," *New York Times*, April 11, 2004.

50   *"Infectious diseases," he says, "systematically steal human resources":* "Disease Burden Links Ecology to Economic Growth," *Science Daily*, December 27, 2012.

50   *"Such a catalog of illnesses!":* Nancy Koehn, "From Calm Leadership, Lasting Change," *New York Times*, October 27, 2012.

55   *"We have never been human":* Donna Haraway, *When Species Meet* (Minneapolis: University of Minnesota Press, 2008), 165.

57–58   *variolation:* Donald Hopkins, *The Greatest Killer: Smallpox in History* (Chicago: University of Chicago Press, 1983,

... 2002), 247–50; Arthur Allen, *Vaccine: The Controversial Story of Medicine's Greatest Lifesaver* (New York: Norton, 2007), 25–33, 46–49.

60 *conference on "immunosemiotics"*: Eli Sercarz et al., *The Semiotics of Cellular Communication in the Immune System* (Berlin: Springer Verlag, 1988), v–viii, 25, 71.

61–62 *When the anthropologist ... vigilance of a mother*: Emily Martin, *Flexible Bodies: Tracking Immunity in American Culture—from the Days of Polio to the Age of AIDS* (Boston: Beacon, 1994), 96, 75, 4.

62–63 *immune system overview*: Thomas Kindt et al., *Kuby Immunology*, 6th ed. (New York: W. H. Freeman, 2007), 1–75.

67 *"children are expected to survive to adulthood"*: Ellen Clayton et al., "Adverse Effects of Vaccines: Evidence and Causality," Institute of Medicine, 2011.

73–76 *women and medicine*: Barbara Ehrenreich and Deirdre English, *For Her Own Good: Two Centuries of the Experts' Advice to Women* (New York: Anchor Books, 1978, 2005), 37–75, 51.

74–75 *Modesty and tradition ... doctors blamed it on tight petticoats, fretting, and bad morals*: Tina Cassidy, *Birth: The Surprising History of How We Are Born* (New York: Grove, 2006), 27–41, 56–59.

75 *Even now ... "it must be maternal"*: Janna Malamud Smith, "Mothers: Tired of Taking the Rap," *New York Times*, June 10, 1990.

75–76 *Wakefield*: Andrew Wakefield et al., "Ileallymphoid-nodular Hyperplasia, Non-Specific Colitis, and Pervasive Developmental Disorder in Children," *Lancet*, February 28, 1998; Editors of the *Lancet*, "Retraction: Ileal Lymphoid Nodular Hyperplasia, Non-specific Colitis, and Pervasive Developmental Disorder in Children," *Lancet*, February 6, 2010; Brian Deer, "MMR—The Truth Behind the Crisis," *Sunday Times*, February 22, 2004; *General Medical Council*, "Fitness to Practise Panel Hearing," January 28, 2010; Cassandra Jardine, "Dangerous Maverick or Medical Martyr?" *Daily Telegraph*, January 29, 2010; Clare Dyer, "Wakefield Was Dishonest and

... Irresponsible over MMR Research, says GMC," *BMJ*, January 2010.

76 *"repeatedly breached fundamental principles of research medicine"* ... *"in particular the association parents made with the vaccine"*: Sarah Boseley, "Andrew Wakefield Struck Off Register by General Medical Council," *Guardian*, May 24 2010.

78 *any number of contagious diseases were caused by bad air ... also for immorality:* Peter Baldwin, "How Night Air Became Good Air: 1776–1930," *Environmental History*, July 2003.

79 *"He was too pure":* Emily Martin, *Flexible Bodies: Tracking Immunity in American Culture—from the Days of Polio to the Age of AIDS* (Boston: Beacon, 1994), 203.

80 *Our breast milk ... "DDT residues and PCBs":* Florence Williams, "Toxic Breast Milk?" *New York Times*, January 9, 2005.

81 *"biologicals of unknown toxicity" ... "cumulative toxic effects":* Jason Fagone, "Will This Doctor Hurt Your Baby?" *Philadelphia Magazine*, June 2009; Barbara Loe Fisher, "NVIC Says IOM Report Confirms Order for Mercury-Free Vaccines," nvic.org, October 1, 2001; Barbara Loe Fisher, "Thimerosal and Newborn Hepatitis B Vaccine," nvic.org, July 8, 1999.

87 *"If you want to understand any moment" ... "modern vampires are not talking as much about sex as they are about power":* Margot Adler, "For the Love of Do-Good Vampires: A Bloody Book List," National Public Radio, February 18, 2010.

89 *The smallpox virus ... "gives the virus its own kind of immortality":* Carl Zimmer, *A Planet of Viruses* (Chicago: University of Chicago Press, 2011), 85–87.

90 *the Polio Pioneers ... allowed them to "request" to be part of the trial:* Jane S. Smith, *Patenting the Sun: Polio and the Salk Vaccine* (New York: Morrow, 1990), 158–59.

91–92 *The polio eradication campaign in Nigeria ... produced by a company based in a Muslim country:* Maryam Yahya, "Polio Vaccines—'No Thank You!': Barriers to Polio Eradication in Northern Nigeria," *African Affairs*, April 2007.

91–93   *polio in Nigeria and Pakistan:* Jeffrey Kluger, "Polio and Politics," *Time*, January 14, 2013; Declan Walsh, "Taliban Block Vaccinations in Pakistan," *New York Times*, June 19, 2012; Maryn McKenna, "File under WTF: Did the CIA Fake a Vaccination Campaign?" Superbug: Wired Science Blogs, wired.com, July 13, 2011 (http://www.wired.com /wiredscience/2011/07/wtf-fake-vaccination/); Donald McNeil, "CIA Vaccine Ruse May Have Harmed the War on Polio," *New York Times*, July 10, 2012; Svea Closser, "Why We Must Provide Better Support for Pakistan's Female Frontline Health Workers," *PLOS Medicine*, October 2013; Aryn Baker, "Pakistani Polio Hits Syria, Proving No Country Is Safe Until All Are," Time.com, November 14, 2013.

95   *Minamata:* Seth Mnookin, *The Panic Virus: A True Story of Medicine, Science, and Fear* (New York: Simon & Schuster, 2011), 120–22.

95–97   *thimerosal:* Walter Orenstein et al., "Global Vaccination Recommendations and Thimerosal," *Pediatrics*, January 2013.

95–96   *"significant reversal" … "profound differences":* Louis Cooper et al., "Ban on Thimerosal in Draft Treaty on Mercury: Why the AAP's Position in 2012 Is So Important," *Pediatrics*, January 2013.

96–97   *"There is no credible scientific evidence" … as global health researchers would observe in* Pediatrics: Katherine King et al., "Global Justice and the Proposed Ban on Thimerosal-Containing Vaccines," *Pediatrics*, January 2013.

99   *"false pandemic":* Fiona Macrae, "The 'False' Pandemic: Drug Firms Cashed in on Scare over Swine Flu, Claims Euro Health Chief," dailymail.co.uk, January 17, 2010.

100   *"Criticism is part of an outbreak cycle":* Jonathan Lynn, "WHO to Review Its Handling of the H1N1 Flu Pandemic," Reuters, January 12, 2010.

100   *In reading the report … "core public-health ethos to prevent disease and save lives":* "Report of the Review Committee on the Functioning of the International Health Regulations (2005) in Relation to Pandemic (H1N1)

... 2009," World Health Organization, May 5, 2011.

101 *"Like capital, Dracula is impelled towards a continuous growth":* Franco Moretti, "The Dialectic of Fear," *New Left Review,* November 1982.

102 *The death toll calculated by the CDC:* F. S. Dawood et al., "Estimated Global Mortality Associated with the First 12 Months of 2009 Pandemic Influenza A H1N1 Virus Circulation: A Modelling Study," *Lancet Infectious Diseases,* June 26, 2012.

103 *"If the White man really wanted to destroy us, there are many other easier ways to do it. They can poison our coca-cola...":* Maryam Yahya, "Polio Vaccines—'No Thank You!': Barriers to Polio Eradication in Northern Nigeria," *African Affairs,* April 2007.

104–110 *paternalism and maternalism:* Michael Merry, "Paternalism, Obesity, and Tolerable Levels of Risk," *Democracy & Education* 20, no. 1, 2012; John Lee, "Paternalistic, Me?" *Lancet Oncology,* January 2003; Barbara Peterson, "Maternalism as a Viable Alternative to the Risks Imposed by Paternalism. A Response to 'Paternalism, Obesity, and Tolerable Levels of Risk,'" *Democracy & Education* 20, no. 1, 2012; Mark Sagoff, "Trust Versus Paternalism," *American Journal of Bioethics,* May 2013.

105 *"If you keep telling people that it's just a marketplace ... in the face of consumer demand.":* Paul Offit, *Do You Believe in Magic? The Sense and Nonsense of Alternative Medicine* (New York: Harper, 2013), 249.

112–115 *"Dr. Bob's Selective Vaccine Schedule" ... "which side effects are truly vaccine related":* Robert Sears, *The Vaccine Book: Making the Right Decision for Your Child* (New York: Little, Brown, 2011), 259, 225, 58, 77; Robert Sears, *The Vaccine Book: Making the Right Decision for Your Child* (New York: Little, Brown, 2007), 57.

112–114 *measles:* Seth Mnookin, *The Panic Virus: A True Story of Medicine, Science, and Fear* (New York: Simon & Schuster, 2011), 19.

114 *It was under Dr. Bob's care that he was not vaccinated:* Seth Mnookin, "Bob Sears: Bald-Faced Liar, Devious

... Dissembler, or Both?" *The Panic Virus: Medicine, Science, and the Media* (blog), PLOS.org, March 26, 2012.

114   *"I was NOT the pediatrician who saw the measles patient"*: Robert Sears, "California Bill AB2109 Threatens Vaccine Freedom of Choice," *Huff Post San Francisco, The Blog* (comments section), March 24, 2012, http:// www.huffingtonpost.com/social/hp_blogger_ Dr.%20Bob20Sears/california-vaccination-bill_b_1355370_143503103.html.

114   *"I have simply been the family's pediatrician"*: Robert Sears, "California Bill AB2109 Threatens Vaccine Freedom of Choice," *Huff Post San Francisco, The Blog* (comments section), March 25, 2012, http://www.huffingtonpost. com /social/hp_blogger_Dr.%20Bob%20Sears/ california-vaccination-bill_b_1355370_143586737.html.

117   *"I will hang you by your neck until you are dead!"*: Paul Offit, *Autism's False Prophets* (New York: Columbia University Press, 2008), xvii.

119   *"In 2008, Merck's revenue"* and *"The 100,000 number ... It's an awful image"*: Amy Wallace, "An Epidemic of Fear: How Panicked Parents Skipping Shots Endangers Us All," *Wired*, October 19, 2009.

122   *A popular alternative to vaccination ... "what they considered 'the real thing'"*: Nadja Durbach, *Bodily Matters: The Anti-Vaccine Movement in England, 1853–1907* (Durham, NC: Duke University Press, 2005), 20.

123   *"taking immunity into your own hands" ... "vigilante vaccination"*: Donald McNeil, "Debating the Wisdom of 'Swine Flu Parties,'" *New York Times*, May 6, 2009.

124–125   *the term conscientious objector ... the conscience was very difficult to define*: Nadja Durbach, *Bodily Matters: The Anti-Vaccine Movement in England, 1853–1907* (Durham, NC: Duke University Press, 2005), 171–97.

125   *George Washington and inoculation*: Seth Mnookin, *The Panic Virus: A True Story of Medicine, Science, and Fear* (New York: Simon & Schuster, 2011), 27–29.

126   *Early vaccine refusers ... under those laws*: Michael Willrich,

... *Pox: An American History* (New York: Penguin, 2011), 330–36.

126–127   *The only vaccine routinely recommended ... "were not at all uncommon":* Arthur Allen, *Vaccine: The Controversial Story of Medicine's Greatest Lifesaver* (New York: Norton, 2007), 111.

129   *"Can we fault parents ..." and "I also warn them ...":* Robert Sears, *The Vaccine Book: Making the Right Decision for Your Child* (New York: Little, Brown, 2007), 220, 97.

131   *"I am but one body naturally considered ...":* Elizabeth I: *Collected Works*, ed. Leah Marcus, Janel Mueller, and Mary Beth Rose (Chicago: University of Chicago Press, 2000), 52.

131   *The Greeks imagined ... "even while the little bodies are fully contained":* Donna Haraway, *Simians, Cyborgs, and Women* (New York: Routledge, 1991), 7, 253.

132   *"a population of self-interested people can defeat an epidemic":* Steve Bradt, "Vaccine Vacuum," *Harvard Gazette*, July 29, 2010; Feng Fu et al., "Imitation Dynamics of Vaccination Behavior on Social Networks," *Proceedings of the Royal Society B*, January 2011.

133   *Attitudes toward the state ... how she thinks about the other:* James Geary, *I Is an Other: The Secret Life of Metaphor and How It Shapes the Way We See the World* (New York: Harper, 2011), 127–29.

133   *"If thought corrupts language":* George Orwell, "Politics and the English Language," *A Collection of Essays* (Orlando: Mariner Books, 1946, 1970), 167.

137   *"In the fall of 1901, regulation was a controversial idea":* Michael Willrich, *Pox: An American History* (New York: Penguin, 2011), 171.

139   *"The imperilled 'immune system'"... "New Age mysticism":* Michael Fitzpatrick, "Myths of Immunity: The Imperiled 'Immune System' Is a Metaphor for Human Vulnerability," *Spiked*, February 18, 2002.

139   *"Why was the term immune system" ... multiple understandings:*

...   AnneMarie Moulin, "Immunology Old and New: The Beginning and the End" in *Immunology 1930–1980*, ed. Pauline Mazumdar (Toronto: Wall & Thompson, 1989), 293–94.

139–140   *The immune system also gathered significance ... one's health becomes overwhelming:* Emily Martin, *Flexible Bodies: Tracking Immunity in American Culture—from the Days of Polio to the Age of AIDS* (Boston: Beacon, 1994), 122.

143   *"Is the immune system at the heart of a new incarnation of social Darwinism" ... "more refined systems of middle-class or upper-class people":* Emily Martin, *Flexible Bodies: Tracking Immunity in American Culture—from the Days of Polio to the Age of AIDS* (Boston: Beacon, 1994), 235, 229.

144   *"Why target two and a half million innocent newborns and children?":* Barbara Loe Fisher, "Illinois Board of Health: Immunization Rules and Proposed Changes," testimony, nvic.org, March 26, 1998.

145–146   *I read an article ... "six impossible (or at least highly improbable) things before breakfast":* Arthur Allen, "In Your Eye, Jenny McCarthy: A Special Court Rejects Autism-Vaccine Theories," *Slate*, February 12, 2009.

146   *"We live in a media culture":* Maria Popova, "Mind and Cosmos: Philosopher Thomas Nagel's Brave Critique of Scientific Reductionism," brainpickings.org (blog), October 30, 2012, http://www.brainpickings.org/index.php/2012/10/30 /mind-and-cosmos-thomas-nagel/.

148   *A former editor was critical of the retraction:* Scott Rosenberg, "Salon.com Retracts Vaccination Story, but Shouldn't Delete It," *Idea Lab* (blog), pbs.org, January 24, 2011, http://www.pbs.org/idealab/2011/01/saloncom-retracts-vaccination-story-but-shouldnt-delete-it021/.

148   *"What matters is the totality of the evidence":* John Ioannidis, "Why Most Published Research Findings Are False," *PLOS Medicine*, August 2005.

149   *"Any science may be likened to a river":* Rachel Carson, *Silent Spring* (New York: Houghton Mifflin, 2002, 1962), 279.

151   *"One can see the insistence throughout the text":* Allan Johnson, "Modernity and Anxiety in Bram Stoker's Dracula," in *Critical Insights: Dracula,* ed. Jack Lynch (Hackensack, NJ: Salem Press, 2009), 74.

156   *"When all was said and done":* Robert Sears, *The Vaccine Book: Making the Right Decision for Your Child* (New York: Little, Brown, 2011), 123.

157   *"The idea of preventive medicine is faintly un-American":* Nicholas von Hoffman, "False Front in War on Cancer," *Chicago Tribune,* February 13, 1975.

158   *"Life":* Donna Haraway, *Simians, Cyborgs, and Women* (New York: Routledge, 1991), 224.

159   *"If we demonize other people":* Susan Dominus, "Stephen King's Family Business," *New York Times,* July 31, 2013.

160   *Offering incentives for giving, one study concluded, can insult people:* Roland Benabou et al., "Incentives and Prosocial Behavior," *American Economic Review,* December 2006.

163–164   *In the fall of 2009 … "used to treat social maladies, such as prejudice":* J. Y. Huang et al., "Immunizing Against Prejudice: Effects of Disease Protection on Attitudes Toward Out-groups," *Psychological Science,* December 22, 2011.

165   *The introductory article in* Science *begins with the myth:* Stephen J. Simpson and Pamela J. Hines, "Self-Discrimination, a Life and Death Issue," *Science,* April 1, 2002.

166–167   *Danger Model:* Polly Matzinger, "The Danger Model: A Renewed Sense of Self," *Science,* April 12, 2002; Claudia Dreifus, "A Conversation with Polly Matzinger: Blazing an Unconventional Trail to a New Theory of Immunity," *New York Times,* June 16, 1998.

167–168   *"caught in an inescapable network of mutuality":* Martin Luther King, "Letter from Birmingham Jail," April 16, 1963.

168   *The article where I learned this:* Carl Zimmer, "Tending the Body's Microbial Garden," *New York Times*, June 18, 2012.

Acknowledgements

Rachel Webster spent many evenings with me, sitting at her kitchen table while our children were sleeping, poring over draft after draft of what would become this book. My writing was fed by conversations with her and other good friends, particularly Suzanne Buffam, Bill Girard, Kristen Harris, Jen Jaume, Amy Leach, Shauna Seliy, Molly Tambor, David Trinidad, and Connie Voisine. Robyn Schiff advised me on all things gothic, thought with me, and articulated things I did not know that I knew. I am grateful to the community of poets— also mothers—who complicated my thinking, argued generously, and pointed me in new directions. I owe particular debts to Brandel France de Bravo, Arielle Greenberg, Joy Katz, Jennifer Kronovet, Cate Marvin, Erika Meitner, Hoa Nguyen, Lisa Olstein, Danielle Pafunda, Martha Silano, Carmen Giménez Smith, Laurel Snyder, Marcela Sulak, and Rachel Zucker, among others.

The writers David Shields and Rebecca Solnit lent me valuable support early in this project. John Keene suggested essential reading on metaphor, and Yiyun Li helped me find an immunologist with a taste for literature. Matt McGowan, my agent, read early drafts of this book and encouraged me to think of it as big even though it was small. My editor, Jeff Shotts, talked out every detail with me and, in his brilliant way, found many opportunities to make this book better. I am grateful to him and everyone at Graywolf.

Grants from the Guggenheim Foundation, the Howard Foundation, and the National Endowment for the Arts allowed me to take time away from teaching for research and writing. The Christine Center provided me with a hermitage. Juthamas Latourte, Aimee Patke Kubes, and our wonderful friends at Total Child Preschool expanded my son's world while I wrote.

Charlotte Cubbage at Northwestern University

Library advised my early research attempts, and
Maria Hlohowskyj served as my first research assistant.
Later, my former student Yliana Gonzalez took time
away from her own writing to assist me—she made this
a smarter book.

The scientists and doctors who generously answered
my many questions include Scott Masten, Ellen Wright
Clayton, Patricia Winokur, Charles Grose, and Paul
Offit. Leonard Green graciously reviewed a full
draft of the book. Tom Waldshmidt explained many
complicated things to me, read through several drafts,
and was an indispensable adviser.

I am grateful to my colleagues at Northwestern for
their ideas and support, particularly Brian Bouldrey,
Katy Breen, Averill Curdy, Nick Davis, Harris
Feinsod, Reg Gibbons, Mary Kinzie, Susan Manning,
Susie Phillips, and Carl Smith. Thanks to Jane
Smith for articulating the problem of power and
powerlessness. Thanks to Laurie Zoloth for introducing
me to bioethics, and for a thrilling discussion of
"Contagion and the Limits of Irony."

Maggie Nelson gave the first full draft of this book
the good, tough read it needed. Nick Davis poured his
brilliance into the margins and buoyed my spirits.
Portions of this book were published in *Harper's*,
and Genevieve Smith made some enduring edits.
Suzanne Buffam, John Bresland, Sarah Manguso,
Mara Naselli, and Robyn Schiff all read drafts and
made valuable suggestions that brought this book to
completion.

I am grateful to my mother, Ellen Graf, for, among
other things, educating me in myth and metaphor. And
to my father, Roger Biss, for nurturing my interest in
immunity, sending me articles, and lending his voice
to this book. My sister Mavis Biss was my companion
in thought, as always, and applied her rigorous mind
to my problems. I am grateful for the many kindnesses
of Cathy Biss, Fred Graf, Athan Biss, Genevieve Biss,

Paroda Decavallas, Liz Graf Brennen, and Louise Langsner.

Thanks to my husband, John Bresland, for collaboratingwith me in life and art, and for being a model of both skepticism and trust. And thanks to my son, Juneau, for giving me so much to think about.